ALLEN CARR

With John Dicey

EASY WAY TO QUIT VAPING

ARCTURUS

ARCTURUS

This edition published in 2021 by Arcturus Publishing Limited
26/27 Bickels Yard, 151–153 Bermondsey Street,
London SE1 3HA, UK

ISBN: 978-1-3988-0045-8
AD008330UK

Printed in the UK

MIX
Paper from
responsible sources
FSC® C018072

ALLEN CARR
With John Dicey

EASY WAY
TO QUIT
VAPING

ALLEN CARR

Allen Carr was a chain-smoker for over 30 years. In 1983, after countless failed attempts to quit, he went from 60–100 cigarettes a day to zero without suffering withdrawal pangs, without using willpower, and without putting on weight. He realised that he had discovered what the world had been waiting for – the easy way to stop smoking – and embarked on a mission to help cure the world's smokers.

As a result of the phenomenal success of his method, he gained an international reputation as the world's leading expert on stopping smoking and his network of centres now spans the globe. His first book, *Allen Carr's Easy Way to Stop Smoking*, has sold over 17 million copies, remains a global bestseller, and has been published in more than 40 different languages. Hundreds of thousands of smokers have successfully quit at Allen Carr's Easyway centres where, with a success rate of over 90 per cent, it's guaranteed you'll find it easy to stop or your money back.

Allen Carr's brilliant Easyway method has been successfully applied to weight control, alcohol, debt, refined sugar, and a host of other addictions and issues.

For more information about Allen Carr's Easyway, please

visit **www.allencarr.com**

Allen Carr's Easyway

The key that will set you free

CONTENTS

Introduction...8

Chapter 1 WHAT'S YOUR POISON?...17

Chapter 2 WHY DO YOU VAPE?... 27

Chapter 3 THE NICOTINE TRAP 41

Chapter 4 THE MYTH 53

Chapter 5 FIRST STEPS TO FREEDOM................................... 65

Chapter 6 THE ILLUSION OF PLEASURE 77

Chapter 7 BELIEF NOT WILLPOWER....................................... 95

Chapter 8 ADDICTIVE PERSONALITY THEORY.................... 105

Chapter 9 CONQUERING CONCENTRATION........................ 113

Chapter 10 SPREADING THE MYTH 135

Chapter 11 SUBSTITUTES DON'T WORK 149

Chapter 12 ARE YOU WORRIED ABOUT YOUR WEIGHT?..... 169

Chapter 13 THE ADVANTAGES OF VAPING 179

Chapter 14 ALL VAPERS ARE THE SAME............................. 181

Chapter 15 VAPING QUESTIONS.. 193

Chapter 16 THE BIGGEST MOMENT OF YOUR LIFE............. 211

Chapter 17 TAKING CONTROL...227

Chapter 18 THE TRUTH ABOUT WITHDRAWAL.....................237

Chapter 19 YOUR FINAL DOSE OF NICOTINE 257

Chapter 20 STAY FREE...267

IT'S IMPORTANT THAT YOU DON'T SKIP THIS IMPORTANT

INTRODUCTION

BY JOHN DICEY, GLOBAL CEO & SENIOR THERAPIST, ALLEN CARR'S EASYWAY

Welcome to *Allen Carr's Easy Way to Quit Vaping*. Allen Carr's reputation in the field of addiction treatment was built on his huge success in helping smokers to quit. His Easyway method was so successful that it quickly became, and remains, a global phenomenon. From the earliest days of Easyway Allen was inundated with requests from victims of countless other addictions and issues, imploring him to apply his method to them. By the turn of the century he had assembled a team of bright, loyal and dedicated senior therapists, who not only helped him to apply the method to all those addictions and issues but also played a key role in delivering Allen Carr's Easyway method across the globe.

The responsibility for ensuring our books are faithful to Allen Carr's original method is mine and it's an honour to be writing this important introduction. Rest assured, once you've read it, I'll leave you in Allen's capable hands. It has been suggested to me that I describe myself as the author of the books we've published since Allen passed away. In my view that would be quite wrong.

That's because every new book is written strictly in accordance with Allen Carr's brilliant Easyway method. In our new books, we have merely updated and amended the format to bring it up to date and make it as relevant as possible for the modern-day audience. There is not a word in our books that Allen didn't write or wouldn't have written if he was still with us and, for that reason, the updates, anecdotes and analogies that are not his own work – that were contemporised or added by me – are written clearly in Allen's voice to seamlessly complement the original text and method.

I consider myself privileged to have worked very closely with Allen on Easyway books while he was alive, gaining insight into how the method could be applied, and we explored and mapped out its future evolution together. I was more than happy to have the responsibility for continuing this vital mission placed on my shoulders by Allen himself. It's a responsibility I accepted with humility and one I take extremely seriously.

The method is as pure, as bright, as adaptable and as effective as it's ever been, allowing us to apply it to a whole host of addictions and guide those who need help in a simple, relatable, plain-speaking way. I know from happy experience that the benefits of following this method can be life-changing.

WHAT ARE OUR CREDENTIALS?

We've been treating nicotine addicts all over the world with phenomenal success over the past 35 years. Whether they be smokers, dippers, nicotine gum chewers or snusers – the method has enabled them to be set free from their addiction. Over the past five years we have also been treating vape addicts, with equal success.

We have provided a money-back guarantee to smokers at our centres for over 35 years and, when we started treating vape addiction at our live seminars, we were so confident in the programme we'd created that we even offered the same money-back guarantee to e-cigarette, tank and JUUL addicts. If they didn't quit nicotine, we'd refund their fee in full.

The refund rate at our live seminars is less than 5 per cent and we continue to offer the money-back guarantee to this day. There are a whole host of eye-wateringly expensive rehab treatment centres around the world, yet we remain, to our knowledge, the only provider of addiction services that provides any form of money-back guarantee. How can we do that?

SIMPLE: THIS METHOD WORKS!

The motivation to write the book was to enable anyone, anywhere in the world, regardless of their level of wealth or poverty, to benefit from *Allen Carr's Easy Way to Quit Vaping*. This isn't simply a transcript of our live seminars – they're dynamic, interactive and last 5–6 hours – but it is certainly the next best thing.

Make no mistake – this is a complete course in itself. While you are reading this book you'll receive all the information you need to set yourself free from nicotine. More importantly than simply being set free, you'll stay free and you'll find it ridiculously easy. That's the whole point of Easyway.

DON'T WORRY IF YOU FEEL SCEPTICAL OR NEGATIVE

No doubt, at this stage, you probably find that a little hard to believe, but don't worry about that – scepticism is a good thing, a great tool – and I'll be asking you to deploy it throughout this book. Not just about everything you read on these pages – but about everything you've been led to believe about nicotine. You might be surprised to learn that virtually everything you think you know about nicotine is actually the opposite of the truth. Hold that thought. I'll return to it in a while.

WHAT WE'RE <u>NOT</u> GOING TO DO IN THIS BOOK

If you're expecting dull and boring details of how the latest nicotine delivery devices (including vaping and heat-not-burn) function technically, with diagrams of heating coils, tank systems or JUUL components and rambling dissertations on ingredients, mods, pods, freebase or salt, I have good news for you. We're not even going to touch on that. Likewise, if you're expecting gory, scary, alarmist details of how dangerous the devices or the ingredients are, and what damage they're likely to do to your lungs, heart and brain, you can rest easy – Allen Carr's Easyway method is unique in that it doesn't attempt to use scare tactics or worries about health to cure addicts.

Don't misunderstand me – if those tactics worked we'd be obliged to utilise them, but the simple truth is that scare tactics don't work. In fact, fear is something that keeps addicts hooked rather than something that inspires them to get free. After all, if you start talking to a vaper or smoker or any other kind of nicotine addict about the terrible health dangers of their addiction, what's the first thing they'll do? They'll close their ears and reach for the drug. A nicotine addict's reaction to fear is to immediately seek out a dose of the drug that causes it.

We're also not interested in the debate about whether e-cigarettes are safer than smoking or not. Who cares about that? The fact is – you want to get free from nicotine addiction, it's your sole objective in buying this book, and there's nothing to be achieved by the smoking versus vaping debate.

Whether you're someone who is addicted to e-cigarettes, JUUL, tanks or pens, any kind of mod or pod (large or small or IQOS or other heat-not-burn devices), nicotine gum, dip, snus or whatever the latest nicotine delivery device is, this method will work for you. In fact, this method will work for addicts of nicotine in any form. If you're someone who combines vaping or other nicotine products AND smoking, known as a dual-user, then this method will certainly work for you – you just need to forgive the fact that most of the language is aimed at smokeless nicotine addicts.

Now, I am going to ask those who exclusively use smokeless nicotine products to indulge me for a minute or two while I provide an overview of the Easyway method and how it was discovered. I promise I won't keep referring to cigarettes or smoking, but at this point it's important that you understand the basis of the method. Afterwards, I'll only reference smoking occasionally and only when it might be useful to do so.

For more than 30 years Allen Carr chain-smoked 60–100 cigarettes a day. He'd tried all the conventional methods to quit smoking and all kinds of substitutes and gimmicks, but nothing worked.

As he described it: 'It was like being between the devil and the deep blue sea, I desperately wanted to quit but whenever I tried I was utterly miserable. No matter how long I survived I never felt completely free – it was as if I'd lost my best friend, my crutch, my character, my very personality. In those days I really believed that there were such types as addictive personalities or that there was something in our genes that meant we couldn't enjoy life or cope with stress without the drug.'

Maybe that sounds familiar or resonates with you?

Eventually, after countless failed attempts to quit, Allen gave up even trying to stop and resigned himself to a lifetime of slavery. Then he discovered something that motivated him to try again. He said:

'I went overnight from a hundred cigarettes a day to zero, without any bad temper or sense of loss, void or depression. On the contrary, I actually enjoyed the process.'

It didn't take Allen long to realise that he had discovered a method which could enable any smoker to quit, easily and immediately, without feeling deprived, without using willpower, substitutes or other gimmicks, without suffering depression or unpleasant withdrawal symptoms and without gaining weight.

After trying out the method on smoking friends and relatives with spectacular success, he gave up his successful career in the financial world to devote himself to helping other smokers quit.

He called the method EASYWAY and it has been a global success story, with centres in more than 150 cities in more than 50 countries worldwide. Bestselling books based on his method are now translated into more than 40 languages, with more being added each year.

It quickly dawned on Allen that the method could be applied to any form of drug addiction. It has helped tens of millions of people quit smoking, vaping, alcohol, cocaine, cannabis, opioids and sugar addiction and achieve freedom from weight issues and even junk spending, caffeine addiction, smart phone addiction, and the fear of flying.

Make no mistake – this isn't a case of Allen Carr's Easyway being a jack of all trades but the master of none. It is THE master. Of all addictions.

HOW DOES IT WORK?

The method works by removing the sense of deprivation that addicts suffer when they try to quit with other methods. It removes the feeling that you are making a sacrifice. This book applies the same method to the issue of vape addiction and, unlike other methods you may have tried, it doesn't rely on willpower.

TOO GOOD TO BE TRUE?

As I mentioned earlier, that might all sound too good to be true. But I assure you, all you have to do is read this book in its entirety and follow all of the instructions, and you will then be set free from your addiction to nicotine.

I'm aware that many people who are unfamiliar with the method, or who have never met people who have successfully used it, assume that some of the claims made about it are far-fetched or exaggerated. That was certainly my reaction when I first heard them.

When I was a chain-smoker my attitude was, 'Sure, quitting would be nice, but I don't have the time right now and since I've tried every quit-smoking method under the sun without any success at all, what's the point in even trying?'

I led a busy life, I had a successful career, and dealing with the pressures those bring, I felt that cigarettes kept me going as a kind of stimulant, that they were a tool which alleviated stress, helped me to relax, helped me to concentrate, and acted as a treat or reward which punctuated my day (as a chain-smoker that was pretty much every 10 minutes!). I was completely convinced that, in spite of the obvious disadvantages of smoking, I was incapable of living my life without cigarettes. Like many smokers who consider themselves 'hopeless cases', I'd settled for what I considered to be a short happy life as a smoker rather than what I considered to be a longer miserable life as a non-smoker. My view was, 'Even if I did manage to quit – what's the point? Who wants to be miserable for the rest of their life?'

I was very fortunate that somebody did eventually hold the truth up for me to see. Twenty or so years ago, I attended Allen Carr's original centre in London, England. I was almost defiant in my disbelief that he might be able to help me quit my 80-a-day smoking addiction. I actually attended under duress. I had agreed to go, at the request of my wife, on the understanding that when I walked out of the seminar still a confirmed smoker she would wait at least 12 months before nagging me about quitting again. No one was more surprised or delighted than I (or perhaps my wife) that Allen Carr's Easyway method set me free.

I was so inspired by Allen and what I saw as his miraculous method that I hassled and harangued him and Robin Hayley (now chairman of Allen Carr's Easyway) to let me get involved in their quest to cure the world of smoking. Thankfully, I succeeded in convincing them. Being trained by Allen and Robin was one of the most rewarding experiences of my life. To be able to count Allen as not only my coach and mentor but also as my friend was an amazing privilege.

Over the past 20 years, I have personally treated more than 30,000 smokers at Allen's original centre in London as well as smokers throughout the USA and in every corner of the globe. It's been my honour to lead the team that has taken his method from London to New York to Mexico City, from Los Angeles to Moscow, from Milwaukee to Singapore, to Sydney, to Santiago and beyond. The book you are holding contains the most up-to-date, cutting edge version of Allen's method specifically to your issue: vape addiction.

Having worked on Allen's books for over 20 years, I still take pleasure (quite rightly) deflecting the praise and acclaim straight back to the great man himself: it's all down to Allen Carr.

I know from happy experience that the benefits of following this method are life-changing. And now let me pass you into the safest of hands – Allen Carr and his Easyway.

Chapter 1

WHAT'S YOUR POISON?

IN THIS CHAPTER
• THIS METHOD IS DIFFERENT   • THE INSTRUCTIONS
• YOU ARE NOT ALONE   • KEEP ON VAPING

Whatever form of nicotine you take, regardless of whether you JUUL it, IQOS it, vape it or take it in any other smokeless fashion – this book will set you free. Most of the time, for clarity and brevity's sake, I'll refer to 'vaping', 'being a vaper' and 'vape addiction' as general terms for your condition, rather than continuously refer to JUUL-addict or IQOS-addict or dip or snus or whatever device or nicotine product you might use. Please don't let that get in the way if you are not a vaper – hopefully you'll understand that it's not possible to refer to each and every form of nicotine delivery system throughout.

IT'S GOING TO BE EASY

Most vape addicts are convinced that it's difficult to quit. The problem, we're told, is not only the physical withdrawal but also that we have to use willpower to resist the craving.

The brilliant news is that you don't have to use willpower, suffer bad withdrawal pangs or use substitutes and you don't have to feel deprived or be left with a feeling of huge sacrifice. If you've tried to quit vaping in the past and failed, if you've battled feelings of deprivation and sacrifice and ended up eventually succumbing to temptation and falling back into the addiction, please put those unhappy experiences behind you.

THIS METHOD IS DIFFERENT

We're going to address the task from an entirely different angle. I'm not going to bang on about the downsides of the addiction; the physical harm, the cost, the slavery, the shame, the low self-esteem, the feelings of hopelessness, the feelings of weakness, the feeling that you aren't quite 'you' any more. That would be patronising and pointless. If those factors were going to help you get free from this addiction, you wouldn't be reading this book now – you know all about that stuff already. Rather than use those downsides in an attempt to motivate yourself to freedom, I want you to ignore them. *Once you're free, release from them simply becomes a wonderful bonus.*

Instead – we're going to ignore the downsides and answer this pertinent question:

'WHAT'S SO GREAT ABOUT BEING A VAPER?'

More about that later...

In the meantime, rest assured, you're on a well-trodden path – more than 50 million people have used Allen Carr's Easyway. They didn't come across the method as a result of multimillion-dollar marketing and advertising campaigns, they came across it as a result of the oldest and most reliable means of referral – what used to be called 'word of mouth'.

Thirty-five years ago it was a slightly slower, more cumbersome process. Someone would try the method, be freed from their addiction and tell their family, friends and colleagues of their success. Those family members, friends and colleagues saw the evidence with their own eyes. These people weren't suffering, they weren't hiding away fearful that they might fall back into the addiction – in fact they simply appeared to have carried on enjoying life, handling stress, relaxing, socialising, having fun and coping with the ups and downs of life without showing the slightest interest in taking the drug again. It didn't matter whether it was nicotine, alcohol, cocaine, sugar or any other drug; the effect was the same – freedom. It was literally word of mouth that carried news of Allen Carr's Easyway method across the globe in those early days; well before the birth of the internet, social media or digital marketing. It became a global phenomenon at breakneck speed the 'old-fashioned way'.

Of course – more recently – word of mouth has become even speedier and more effective; with social media, bloggers and instant communication, good news travels faster than ever. In fact, it's quite likely that the reason you're reading this, the means by which you originally discovered Allen Carr's Easyway, was via a member of your family, a friend or a colleague telling you about their own success with the method.

NOW IT'S YOUR TURN. GET SET TO BE FREE FROM VAPING

Let this be the first stage of an exciting adventure; the moment you start preparing yourself to be free. All you need to do is follow the instructions given.

YOUR FIRST INSTRUCTION IS:
YOU MUST FOLLOW ALL OF THE INSTRUCTIONS

You could spend a lifetime trying to break into a safe and still not succeed. But if you know the correct combination to the lock, or if you have the key, it's ridiculously easy. Forget one number in the combination or lose the key and you'll remain trapped.

This book contains the key, the combination of information you need in order to become free. It will enable you to escape from nicotine addiction. Follow the instructions I give you and you will succeed. Ignore one of them and you jeopardise your entire objective.

YOUR SECOND INSTRUCTION IS: DON'T ATTEMPT TO CUT DOWN
OR CONTROL YOUR VAPING UNTIL I ADVISE YOU TO DO SO

I will ask you to stop vaping towards the end of this book.

Of course, if you have already abstained for a few days there is no need to carry on vaping, but if you want to vape – do so. Vape as normal, even while you are reading the book. I don't want you to be using willpower to resist the inclination to vape, as doing so before you've come to the end of the book is likely to interfere with the method's success.

TO FIND IT EASY TO QUIT VAPING YOU MUST ACHIEVE A FRAME OF MIND WHEREBY ANY TIME YOU THINK ABOUT VAPING OR NICOTINE IN ANY FORM, YOU FEEL A SENSE OF RELEASE, FREEDOM AND RELIEF BECAUSE YOU DON'T CONSUME IT ANY MORE. THAT REALLY IS THE ONLY WAY TO BECOME, AND REMAIN, TRULY FREE AND NO LONGER VULNERABLE TO THE DRUG.

Changing, or more accurately correcting, your perception of vaping and nicotine will actually be an exciting, eye-opening and positive experience. Although you might find that hard to believe, you have absolutely nothing to lose and everything to gain by accepting that it's going to be exactly that way.

YOUR THIRD INSTRUCTION IS: START OFF IN A HAPPY FRAME OF MIND

This is closely followed by the fourth instruction:

YOUR FOURTH INSTRUCTION IS: THINK POSITIVELY

Cast aside all feelings of impending doom and gloom. Nothing bad is going to happen and there is no need to be miserable or anticipate failure or difficulty. You're about to achieve something truly marvellous, something amazing. See your short journey through this book as it really is – an exciting challenge. An adventure. Just think how proud you'll feel when you're free. If you vape in secret, this might be a private achievement for you – something that will remain a secret to those who are nearest and dearest to you. But don't let that temper the feeling. You're about to impress the most important person on the planet: YOU!

'HERE'S LOOKING AT YOU KID.'

This book will give you all you need to set yourself free, regardless of your age. When planning this book, I was acutely aware that the age range of the reader would be extremely broad. If you're a youngster reading this, we make no apologies for 'playing it straight' and avoiding a patronising 'young-adult' writing style. You've picked up this book because you have a serious problem – you've become addicted to nicotine – and as you read it you'll find that it imparts the exact information you need, in exactly the way you need it, in order for you to be able to set yourself free.

For the older reader, the fact that, in the early twenty-first century, we've somehow allowed Big Tobacco and Big Pharma to succeed in enslaving our youth in front of our very eyes is not testimony to our weakness or lack of care, but is a measure of the frightening power, obscene determination and political influence of the nicotine industry.

YOUNG OR OLD – THIS IS WHEN YOU FIGHT BACK, THIS IS WHERE YOU TAKE BACK CONTROL, COCKING A SNOOK AT BIG NICOTINE AS YOU WALK TO FREEDOM. ENJOY IT.

You're reading the most up-to-date, cutting edge, best-practice version of *Allen Carr's Easy Way to Quit Vaping* method, which will not only set you free from vaping, JUULing, IQOS, chewing tobacco, dip, snus or any other nicotine product, but will ensure that you find it easy, and even enjoyable.

The fifth instruction is the most difficult to follow:

YOUR FIFTH INSTRUCTION IS: KEEP AN OPEN MIND

I can't overemphasise the importance of keeping an open mind. Some people believe this method is a form of brainwashing. In a way that's a tribute to its effectiveness – but in fact nothing could be further from the truth.

WHAT WE DO IS ACTUALLY COUNTER-BRAINWASHING

If you figuratively imagine brainwashing as, for example, the gradual damaging or over-tightening of a coil or spring, all we do – over the course of a few hours, or during the time it takes you to read this book – is gradually, painlessly and safely stop the unnatural and damaging over-tightening process, and then gently and calmly reverse it. This will eventually leave the coil or spring in its natural, healthy, safe condition. That's counter-brainwashing.

This method involves the reversal of false beliefs that you may have entertained throughout your entire life. You need to question what you think you know about vaping. Question what society, other addicts and even your own experiences have led you to believe about nicotine. If you can do that, and you follow all the other instructions, you cannot fail.

Vapers, like smokers, are notorious for burying their heads in the sand. You can only continue to do something that you know is harmful and degrading if you close your mind to the fact. As a result, nicotine addiction becomes a lonely experience. Ironically, for something that is supposed to be a sociable activity, it leaves vapers feeling as if they have a problem that is unique to them.

But I can tell you now:

YOU ARE NOT ALONE

As you read this book, thousands of other e-cigarette addicts are doing the same thing – trying to find a cure for their nicotine problem.

You *have* taken the crucial first step of opening your mind to the fact that you want to stop vaping, JUULing or being addicted to any other form of nicotine addiction. You have admitted that there is something about nicotine use that makes you unhappy – you may not know exactly what it is yet, but you know it's serious and you want to find a solution. Whether you stumbled across Easyway or, more likely, it was recommended by a friend, colleague or unsolicited celebrity endorsement, be reassured: you're in safe hands, and whether you believe it or not at this point, freedom awaits.

Some people have spent months or even years trying and failing to quit vaping. Others quit in an instant. If you think that's because there are different types of vaper, think again.

All nicotine addicts are caught up in the same trap. I tried and failed on countless occasions before I discovered the method that enabled me to quit permanently.

What changed? It was my understanding of the problem.

Like most nicotine addicts, I believed that it gave me some sort of pleasure or crutch. I believed this, even though I took no pleasure in doing it and it made me feel miserable. I didn't realise that I was being fooled; that I'd simply fallen into the most sinister and subtle trap that man and nature have ever combined to devise. A mixture of brainwashing and addiction had led me to believe that nicotine provided me with something beneficial or pleasurable.

As soon as I saw through the illusion, my desire to use nicotine in any form disappeared and I was able to help other nicotine addicts quit easily, immediately and painlessly, without relying on willpower or substitutes, or having to endure any unpleasant withdrawal feelings. I'm going to spend the initial stage of your journey to freedom looking at your understanding of vaping and why you think you do it. By the end of this stage you will have developed a real understanding of why you vape, why you've been unable to quit until now, how vaping distorts and disrupts your behaviour, and what action you need to take to begin your successful bid for freedom.

ALL YOU HAVE TO DO IS FOLLOW THE INSTRUCTIONS.

KEEP ON VAPING

As mentioned already, there is no need to stop vaping or using any other nicotine product, or to try and change your vaping pattern, until you reach the end of the book. I'll be sure to let you know when that point is approaching. In fact, it's important that you keep on vaping as usual. Don't worry that the idea of carrying on for the time being makes you happy and don't be concerned if the idea of quitting by the end of the book makes you feel nervous or anxious or miserable. Trust that this book will answer every single question and any doubt that you might have. Trust that it will lead you to a new life as a happy non-vaper. You've got nothing to lose from that approach and everything to gain.

Right now, you are still a nicotine addict, so if you feel the urge to vape, go ahead. It's important that you don't do anything that you might interpret as self-deprivation. Don't adjust the nicotine content of your vape – just carry on as you are. I will explain why later on. Likewise, if you haven't vaped for more than a day or so, but remain hooked on nicotine gum or patches or any other nicotine product, carry on using that product as you have done until now – without attempting to cut down or control your use.

For now, all you need to know is that there is no pain when you quit with Easyway. You don't need willpower; you just need to follow the instructions and find out how easy it is to get free from nicotine and, more importantly, stay free.

Chapter 2

WHY DO YOU VAPE?

IN THIS CHAPTER
• MEET NICOTINE • WHAT IS WITHDRAWAL?
• NO WILLPOWER REQUIRED • THE LITTLE MONSTER
• A LOGICAL CONCLUSION • THIS IS GREAT NEWS
• BRAINWASHING

Vapers give all sorts of reasons when asked why they do it. They seldom give the correct answer. So we are going to begin by making sure you're aware of the real reason you vape.

MEET NICOTINE

When you vape, you inhale a drug called nicotine. You could replace the word 'drug' with 'poison'. Let's strip it down and examine it.

In its pure form, nicotine is a colourless, oily compound that is lethal to humans in relatively small doses. It is the fastest-acting addictive drug known to mankind, faster than heroin. Each puff on a JUUL or IQOS or e-cigarette delivers a dose of nicotine to the brain, via the lungs, within just eight seconds – that's faster than a dose of heroin injected directly into the bloodstream.

If you take 20 puffs of vape, then you're taking 20 individual doses or shots. This is like 'machine-gunning' nicotine into your body. Nicotine is quick to enter the system but it is also quick to leave it too. As soon as you put your vape pen down, the nicotine level rapidly subsides and the drug begins to withdraw from your body. If you measured the amount of the drug in your bloodstream after finishing vaping, you would find it had fallen to roughly half after 30 minutes and to about a quarter after an hour. It doesn't matter how much you vape or how little you vape – you'll find it equally easy to stop.

NICOTINE LEAVES THE BODY VERY QUICKLY. WITHIN EIGHT HOURS OF QUITTING VAPING YOU ARE 97 PER CENT NICOTINE-FREE, WITHIN THREE DAYS YOU'RE 100 PER CENT NICOTINE-FREE.

What do you understand by withdrawal?

Most nicotine addicts associate the word with the 'terrible pangs and cravings' they suffer when they try to quit. In fact, the physical symptoms of withdrawal are so slight as to be almost imperceptible. Don't misunderstand me. The unpleasant physical symptoms you suffered when you may have attempted to quit previously are real: they're just not caused by nicotine withdrawal. Instead, they're a physical response to a mental process – of 'wanting a vape' but not being able to have one.

I'll explain more later, but if, just on principle, you can accept that, then you have taken a huge step towards being free already. If you're not sure you can accept that, even in principle, don't panic. Let's look at it in more detail.

THE UNPLEASANT PHYSICAL FEELINGS ARE REAL, BUT THEY ARE THE RESULT OF A MENTAL PROCESS – OF WANTING A VAPE AND NOT BEING ABLE TO HAVE ONE

Think of a child having their favourite toy taken away from them. The physical symptoms it causes are real and measurable: red face, bulging eyes, anger, rage, an anxious, uptight and insecure feeling.

Does that sound familiar? Doesn't it describe the feeling you've had in the past when you've tried to quit without success? But the fact is, the child isn't suffering from the physical withdrawal from a drug; it's simply a selection of physical symptoms, resulting from a mental process: 'I WANT IT! I CAN'T HAVE IT! AGHHHH!'

It's 'wanting a vape' that causes the really unpleasant symptoms when you try to break free from nicotine addiction, rather than it simply being the physical withdrawal from nicotine:

'I WANT A VAPE! I CAN'T HAVE ONE! AGHHHH!'

The physical response to that thought process is that uptight, anxious, churned-up, angry feeling that you identify as physical withdrawal.

The only reason you 'want a vape' is because you believe it will do something positive for you.

Therefore, if I can explain that nicotine in any form does absolutely nothing for you, and furthermore if I can explain how you got fooled into thinking that it did, then you won't want to vape. True?

So let's take it a stage further. If you don't want a vape, then you won't have that 'I WANT A VAPE! I CAN'T HAVE ONE! AGHHHH!' feeling. True?

Now, that's a lot to take in, especially so early on in this process. I don't want you to agree entirely with what I'm saying at this stage. I just want you to consider the possibility that what I am saying is true; I want you to at least have an understanding of where I'm coming from.

NO WILLPOWER REQUIRED

Any real discomfort nicotine addicts experience when they try to quit is mostly mental, as they wrestle with the thought of wanting something they can't have and feel the need to battle the temptation to vape again.

Doesn't this make sense of those ex-vapers, AND ex-smokers, you meet from time to time – the ones who haven't done it for months or even years but are still tearing their hair out? They don't have a trace of nicotine left in their bodies – so there is no physical withdrawal at all – yet they still mope after the drug. It's the 'moping' that causes the unpleasant physical feelings, not nicotine withdrawal.

But *you* won't go through this discomfort. With Easyway, there is no mental struggle. That's why you don't need willpower.

The physical withdrawal from nicotine is so slight most addicts aren't even aware that they suffer it every day, and every night, of their vaping lives. Most of them are never aware of it. It manifests itself as nothing more than a mild, empty, slightly insecure feeling – not unlike hunger – which you interpret as the feeling of 'something's missing'.

Nicotine is an addictive drug that hooks you very quickly – just one e-cigarette is enough – but luckily, it's just as easy to get 'unhooked'. Nicotine leaves your system completely within a few days. Why, then, do addicts find it so hard to quit? And why do vapers and smokers who have not done it for months or even years still crave that nicotine?

THE ADDICTION IS 1 PER CENT PHYSICAL AND 99 PER CENT MENTAL!

Given that is true, can you see how pointless it is to use nicotine products in an attempt to quit being addicted?

E-cigarettes, nicotine patches and gum, nicotine inhalators and lozenges attempt to address just 1 per cent of the problem, leaving you suffering the other 99 per cent – the mental side. No wonder you've failed in the past. Handle the mental side of things and the 1 per cent physical addiction is easy to break.

When we first started helping smokers to escape from the smoking trap, it was actually quite difficult to have them understand that they were addicted.

These are more enlightened times and most smokers and vapers these days are fairly comfortable with the idea that they're addicts. Comfortable is probably the wrong word – no one likes being an addict — but at least these days people are prepared to accept the fact rather than attempt to live in denial.

The issue which remains, though, is the belief that to be addicted to something you have to enjoy it, or get pleasure from it, or get some form of benefit from it.

By the time you finish this book you'll have a clear understanding of how addiction *really* works. And trust me, it has nothing to do with 'liking' the drug, 'enjoying' the drug or getting 'pleasure' or 'benefits' from the drug.

If you began this book unaware that you're addicted, or are reluctant to accept that you are, don't worry. Just carry on reading, assess the evidence and allow yourself to come to a conclusion as you work your way through the book. Nothing bad is going to happen and you don't have to have your final e-cigarette or JUUL or IQOS or other nicotine product until you're happy to do so.

AND I DO MEAN 'HAPPY'

Being an addict can be hard for some nicotine addicts to accept. Vaping is a much more socially acceptable drug than heroin and most vapers prefer to think of it as 'just a habit' they fell into and can't seem to kick, rather than seeing themselves as drug addicts. But the acceptance that you're addicted to nicotine is key to your escape. Seeing yourself as anything but a drug addict will lead to misconceptions about why you vape and what vaping does for you, and it's these misconceptions that keep nicotine addicts in the trap.

Only by recognising that you are an addict can you begin the process of becoming a non-addict again.

An addictive drug like nicotine works in a fiendishly clever way. Within eight seconds of inhaling nicotine, a fresh dose of nicotine is supplied to the brain and the slightly edgy feeling of withdrawal from the previous dose subsides.

This creates the impression of satisfaction, relaxation and confidence, which vapers naturally attribute to nicotine.

Think about that for a moment. Every single time you've inhaled nicotine, every single day of your life as a vaper, you've felt slightly better than the moment before. But all that happened, on every single occasion, is the e-cigarette or JUUL or IQOS momentarily got rid of the unpleasant feeling caused by the previous one. This is the very slight, very mild, feeling of nicotine withdrawal. It's so slight you've been unaware of it for most of your nicotine-addicted life.

In fact, if you were to pay attention to the vape and the way you feel as you prepare to inhale it (very few, if any, vapers do this), you would notice that the edgy feeling ends as soon as you pick up your nicotine device and bring it to your lips. It doesn't take eight seconds. You don't even need to inhale it. You don't need the drug to relieve the withdrawal symptoms; you just need to know that you're about to get it. This goes to show that addiction is not simply a condition of the body but mainly of the mind. Let me repeat what I told you a short while ago: **ADDICTION IS 1 PER CENT PHYSICAL AND 99 PER CENT MENTAL.**

It's your mind that we are working on, making sure you're fully prepared to accept the changes that will lead you to freedom from vaping, freedom from addiction.

When we first start vaping we're not aware of this process of withdrawal and relief because the pangs are so slight that we don't notice them. As vaping becomes a regular part of our life we assume it's because we enjoy it or we've just got into the 'habit'. It doesn't cross our minds that we've become addicted. But when you understand how addiction works, it's easy to accept that you are addicted to nicotine, and that addiction is not driven by genuine pleasure or genuine relief, but is a simple confidence trick.

Imagine someone you think of as a friend who, without your knowledge, was stealing £100 from your bank account. After doing so, imagine they give you £10 to spend on whatever you want. It would appear to be a lovely thing for them to do. They'd appear to be generous and kind. But are they really?

Is the £10 real? Of course it is. How can you view someone giving you £10 as being anything other than kind and generous? It's only when you have all the information – only when you find out that the £10 was already yours and, what's more, that the thief has kept another £90 of yours in their back pocket – that you see the 'gift' of £10, and the so-called friend, as they really are. A sham. A con. A rip-off! If you're thinking, 'Well, at least they gave £10 of the £100 back to me – they could have taken it all,' remember, this thief has been stealing from you like this for years. He doesn't deserve one ounce of gratitude.

THE LITTLE MONSTER

The first vape introduces nicotine into your system for the first time. You put down the JUUL or IQOS or e-cigarette, or whatever device you used, and for the first time, without even realising it, you experience the physical withdrawal from nicotine. It's as if the first vape created a little nicotine monster inside your body, like a tapeworm, that feeds on nicotine.

As the nicotine withdraws from your body, the little nicotine monster expresses its dissatisfaction. It's a mild, empty, insecure feeling, so slight it's almost imperceptible. When you have your next vape, the mild, empty, slightly insecure feeling disappears (you've effectively fed the Little Monster) and you feel slightly better than a moment before. A lifetime's chain has started.

Whatever you may think are your reasons for continuing to vape, there is only one reason: to feed the Little Monster.

You know what it's like when a neighbour's burglar alarm has been ringing all day? You find a way to blot it out so you can get on with other things, but then suddenly the alarm stops and you experience a wonderful sense of relief. The peace feels heavenly, but all you're enjoying is the end of the aggravation. It's the same when a vaper vapes and feeds the Little Monster. All you're trying to do is get rid of the aggravation of nicotine withdrawal. It's an empty, insecure feeling that is hard to pinpoint but nevertheless leaves you feeling slightly out of sorts.

Non-vapers don't suffer from that feeling and neither did you before you started vaping. So why do you do it?

TO FEEL LIKE A NON-VAPER!

Many vapers will argue until they're blue in the face that it gives them pleasure. But the only pleasure you can hope to get from vaping is the feeling of removing the aggravation caused by the Little Monster and restoring the state of calm and confidence that you had before you became addicted. In fact, you can never return to the state of calm and confidence of a non-vaper by vaping.

THE ONLY WAY TO FEEL LIKE A NON-VAPER IS BY NOT VAPING

The great news is that the Little Monster is actually very weak – it's easy to kill. What the Little Monster does, though, is act as a trigger for the Big Monster, a mental process that develops as a result of you appearing to feel better after vaping. The effect of this process, day in, day out, every single day of your vaping life confuses your brain into thinking that nicotine provides some kind of pleasure or crutch. It's like being fooled by the conman who steals £100 from your bank account without your knowledge and then gifts you £10.

Before you started vaping your body was complete. Then you forced nicotine into your body and, as the drug started to leave your body, suffered the slightly restless feeling of withdrawal. It wasn't a physical pain; in fact, it was so slight that you probably didn't consciously register it. Your reaction to it, though, was to have another dose of nicotine.

Time passes by and your conscious mind doesn't understand the feelings or your response to them. All you know is that you want another vape and when you have one the slightly empty feeling goes. Again, you don't really register the feeling going, you just feel a little better; a little more confident and complete than a moment before. In fact, the way you felt was how you felt your whole life before you first vaped. It was nothing more than relieving the aggravation caused by the first vape.

And so it goes on, each vape creating the desire for the next. It's a vicious circle that ties you up for life – unless you break the cycle.

EXERCISE: PAY ATTENTION

Vapers say they enjoy doing it. They insist that they like the taste, the smell, the feeling of it in their hand. In truth, the vast majority of vapes occur without you being aware of the taste, smell, feel or any other aspect of what you're doing.

When you next vape, pay attention to every part of the process. Concentrate on the packet or device – how does it look? What does it look like as you prepare it and lift it to your lips? And how do you feel?

How is your heartbeat? Continue applying this level of attention as you go through your usual routine, placing it between your lips, inhaling that first drag, blowing the vape out of your lungs. As you proceed how does it smell? How does it taste? What is the sensation on your tongue? In your throat? In your nose? In your lungs? How does it look in your hand? As you reach the end put the device down in front of you. How does it look? What taste has it left in your mouth? And how do you feel inside?

I'm not expecting this exercise to put you off vaping. That is not the point. What is important is that you have a clear perception of the truth when it comes to your personal experience of vaping. At the moment, your perception of it is shrouded in a fog of brainwashing. Like all vapers, you assume there must be something marvellous about it that keeps you coming back for more.

Make no mistake, the only reason you come back for more is

---

to feed the Little Monster.

Please be vigilant here; whichever nicotine product or device you use, adapt the exercise accordingly. Only then are you ready to move on. Don't feel under any pressure to draw any conclusions from the exercise – however you feel is perfectly fine. Incidentally, if you haven't vaped for a few days please don't feel obliged to do so. There'll be guidance for you later in the book.

A LOGICAL CONCLUSION

If vaping, JUULing, IQOSing or any other kind of nicotine use is just an addiction, then it follows that you don't do it for pleasure or a crutch, or to help you concentrate or feel more confident. Does a heroin addict inject the drug because it helps him concentrate? Of course not. It's easy to see that a heroin addict continues to take the drug because the addiction makes him feel terrible when he has to go without. There is nothing more complex or sophisticated about it than that. Be careful not to fall for Hollywood's glamourised view of drugs as being the providers of an amazing high. For the most part, someone taking heroin for the first time doesn't feel fabulous or high or amazing; in fact, it's quite the reverse.

So it should be just as easy to see vaping in the same light. You vape to get nicotine. You only want nicotine because you're addicted to it – the Little Monster makes you feel restless and empty without it.

And if addiction to nicotine is the only reason vapers vape, nicotine gum chewers chew, snusers snus or dippers dip, then it doesn't make any difference who the addict is. There is no genetic difference between vapers and non-vapers and there is no difference between different types of vaper. Vaping is simply a trap into which anybody can fall if they have an experimental e-cigarette, JUUL, IQOS or other nicotine product. Because once you've put nicotine in your body, all it takes is the second dose to feed the Little Monster and you begin a lifetime's journey into the nicotine pit.

THIS IS GREAT NEWS

If the only reason you vape is because you're addicted to nicotine, all you need to do to quit is remove the addiction. You don't have to 'give up' anything; there is no sacrifice, no deprivation. You don't need to draw on all your reserves of willpower to resist the temptation to vape because there is no temptation. Neither is there anything in your personality to hold you back. All there is is a gradual descent into addiction, which, you'll be delighted to know, is easy to reverse.

BREAK THE CHAIN AND YOU WILL BE FREE

The real trick, and the one essential to making it easy to not just stop, but to stay stopped – and not just to be a non-vaper, but to be a happy non-vaper – is to truly understand why you thought you got tremendous pleasure, enjoyment and support from taking this drug.

We've dealt with the principle and process of the addiction, the Little Monster; later we'll deal with the brainwashing, the Big Monster. It's the Big Monster that has caused the torture and hell, along with the feelings of deprivation in your previous attempts to quit.

BRAINWASHING

Despite the success of Easyway, nicotine remains the world's number one killer. Working against us is a hugely powerful machine which continues to brainwash people into believing that they choose to vape or smoke because it gives them some sort of pleasure or crutch.

I don't just mean the tobacco industry. Television and films continue to play an influential role in portraying vaping or smoking as something cool, suave and characterful. Every singer or celebrity seen with a cigarette or vape in their mouth is responsible for countless thousands of impressionable fans experimenting with nicotine.

Against this weight of propaganda, how is any nicotine addict expected to see the simple truth?

YOU DO NOT CHOOSE TO VAPE

Think about it – if you had any choice over whether you vape or not, you wouldn't be reading this book. You vape because you are caught in a trap and because if you've tried to quit in the past, you've failed to do so. This time it's going to be different.

Vapers who cannot see and understand this simple truth find it hard to quit. Why? Because they go about it in the wrong way. Follow the right method and quitting is easy. The starting point is understanding why you vape.

Chapter 3

THE NICOTINE TRAP

IN THIS CHAPTER
• *THE PITCHER PLANT* • *SECURITY OF THE PRISON*
• *THE TUG-OF-WAR OF FEAR* • *THE PLEASURE OF VAPING*
• *THE BIG MONSTER* • *YOUR OBJECTIVE*
• *ESCAPE IS EASY*

We've established the real reason why you vape – because you're in a trap called nicotine addiction. Now we need to examine the trap you're in, learn how it works and understand how you can escape.

THE PITCHER PLANT

The more subtle a trap is, the more effective it is at catching unsuspecting victims. The nicotine trap is so ingenious that not only do its victims not see it coming, they don't even realise when they've been caught. It only dawns on them when they're well and truly hooked and struggling to escape.

A good comparison is the pitcher plant, that carnivorous wonder of nature which feeds on flies. The pitcher plant is so-called because of its distinctive jug shape. The plant's nectar attracts flies, which alight on the upper rim of the pitcher and start to feed. The fly has no fear of the plant. Why should it? It can fly off whenever it wants. But right now the nectar tastes good, so there's no reason to think about flying away.

As the fly continues to feed, it ventures deeper into the pitcher. The sides are steeper here and slippery with sweet nectar. The fly loses its grip occasionally and turns back towards the light, but the nectar is too good to resist and the instinct to fly away is not triggered until it's too late. By the time the fly realises that there's something wrong about this plant, it's lost its grip and fallen into the digestive juices at the bottom of the pitcher. Now it's the plant devouring the fly, rather than the other way around.

With the nicotine trap, there is no sweet nectar to lure victims. The lure is purely psychological. We all try our first experimental JUUL, IQOS or e-cigarette for a variety of foolish reasons. From birth we're brainwashed into believing that nicotine use might help us to fit in, appear more grown-up, seem more sophisticated or be rebellious. The list is endless. Regardless of how first-time vapers find the taste and smell, or rate the experience (normally no more than the curiosity and excitement of trying something new), they are still drawn into the trap because somewhere in their mind the seed has been sown that vaping is something that can give them pleasure. They're not exactly sure what that pleasure is – and those first puffs certainly don't offer any insight – but they know enough people who do it to convince them that it's worth the effort.

The underwhelming experience of the first vape is enough to prevent some first-time vapers from ever vaping a second time and thus never getting hooked, but for others it contributes to the deadly lure of the trap.

It makes them think, 'I could never get hooked on this', and so they stumble on, confident that they could stop any time they choose. Like the fly, their confidence is dreadfully misplaced.

SECURITY OF THE PRISON

The nicotine trap is not just ingenious in the way it snares its victims. Even when they realise they're hooked and desperately wish they could escape, the trap grips them tighter, making the idea of escape seem more daunting than the prospect of staying in the trap.

There is a similar psychological effect with long-term convicts when they're finally released from prison. Rather than embracing their newfound freedom, a large proportion of prisoners reoffend within a short period of their release. They don't do it because they believe that crime will pay and they'll get away with it this time; they do it because they want to get caught and put back inside. They crave what they've come to consider the security of the prison.

Prison may be tough, confined and miserable but for the long-term convict it offers the comfort of familiarity. The world outside is daunting and full of questions: Can I fend for myself? How do things work? Will I cope with all the changes? Will anyone want to know me? For vapers, the nicotine trap offers the same feeling of 'security'. This is what grips you and makes it hard to escape. You know that vaping is not healthy, that it's already damaging your health and wealth – and being enslaved and controlled by a drug feels demeaning and embarrassing. In public it feels foolish and unsophisticated to be puffing on the device, not being able to stop, and yet the prospect of living life without vape, and suffering torture and hell in the attempt to get free, puts you off the idea of even trying to quit. On top of that is the assumption that, even if you succeed in quitting, you'll end up feeling miserable and deprived for the rest of your life.

Rather than seeing the nicotine trap as a hellish prison that they want to escape from at the earliest possible opportunity, vapers feel a sense of being trapped between a rock and a hard place.

THE TUG-OF-WAR OF FEAR

The force that drives the long-term prisoner to reoffend so soon after being released is FEAR. Vapers block their minds to the effects of the addiction for the same reason. They perhaps reassure themselves that at least they're not smoking, although often they become ensnared in that trap too – or at least feel tempted. If they paid heed to what their instincts told them about vaping, they would have to stop – and that frightens them even more. This explains why vapers spend their lives blocking their minds to the many powerful reasons to quit and search for any flimsy excuse to have 'just one more' vape.

Nicotine addicts are pulled apart by a constant tug-of-war that takes place in their mind. On one side is the voice saying: 'It's killing me and costing me a fortune. It's filthy, embarrassing and it's controlling my whole life.' And on the other is a voice saying: 'How can I enjoy life and cope with stress without my little pleasure or crutch? Quitting won't be easy. Do I have the willpower to even try? And will I ever be able to say I'm completely free?'

There is one thing at both ends of this tug-of-war: FEAR. It is overwhelmingly fear that keeps nicotine addicts trapped. At one end, the fear of what will happen to us if we carry on vaping – at the other, the fear of what will happen if we stop: how will we cope?

Easyway will get rid of both of those fears. Don't worry, I have no intention whatsoever of preaching to you about the downsides of vaping. You know all about those already – or at least suspect them. The biggest mistake that well-intentioned health campaigns make is to utilise fear to encourage addicts to stop.

Firstly, as vapers we turn a blind eye to it anyway. The moment someone on the radio or TV starts talking about the damage caused by vaping we simply switch channels. Even on those rare occasions that we allow ourselves to dwell on the downsides of the addiction, in situations where we're forced to do so, what's the first thing we do? We suck on a vape. A vaper's reaction to any stressful situation is to vape. Attempting to cure a nicotine addict by telling them about the damage it's causing them is not only an insult to their intelligence, but a complete waste of time; it's entirely counter-productive, like trying to extinguish a fire with a bucket of petrol.

As soon as you're a happy non-vaper, the fear and embarrassment of being an addict disappears. It's a fabulous feeling of freedom. One you can anticipate with relish. Getting rid of the fear on either side of the tug-of-war, the worry about how you'll cope without vaping, how you'll handle stress, how you'll manage to relax, control your weight, enjoy socialising and live everyday life without nicotine is what this book will achieve.

THE PLEASURE OF VAPING

As I demonstrated in the last exercise, most vaping is done without paying any attention. The only times you're aware of it are:

- when your vape cloud is bothering other people

- when you become sick of the smell of whatever vape flavour you're using

- when you feel embarrassed by your need to do it and wish you'd never started

- or when you're in a situation where you're not permitted to vape and you're feeling deprived and miserable because of it.

So what sort of pleasure is that? You're either not aware that you're vaping or you're wishing you weren't, and it only seems precious when you can't do it! Yet vapers are terrified by the prospect of spending the rest of their life without it.

THE BIG MONSTER

The lure of the nicotine trap is purely psychological. Nobody takes up vaping because they are drawn to the taste or smell. Whenever a non-vaper stands somewhere and they're surrounded by a popcorn flavour or candy floss flavour or cucumber or mint or mango flavour vape cloud, they can attest to the fact that, far from smelling alluring, it smells pretty awful. As repulsive to most people as cheap, trashy perfume. It's the belief that they are getting into something a bit naughty or pleasurable, or beneficial, that lures vapers in.

It's the same belief that keeps them trapped. The vaper's tug-of-war of fear exists because of the belief that vaping gives you some sort of pleasure or crutch. Take away that belief and the arguments for doing it simply disappear. Vaping, and any form of nicotine addiction, becomes exposed for what it really is: pointless. And if there is genuinely no point in doing something, why would it require any willpower not to do it? It doesn't. You'll be no more inclined to stick a JUUL or IQOS or e-cigarette in your mouth than you might be to stick it in your ear.

I've introduced you to the Little Monster, which feeds on the nicotine from each vape and complains as the nicotine leaves your system. When you have the next vape, the Little Monster is satisfied and you feel a sense of relief flooding back in. But then it floods back out and the Little Monster starts moaning again. This is the cycle of addiction. Vapers believe that it helps relieve their stress and help them relax and concentrate. They don't realise that it's vaping which causes these problems in the first place.

KILL THE LITTLE MONSTER AND YOU END THE ADDICTION

All you have to do to kill the Little Monster is starve it of nicotine – it dies within a matter of days. That's how long it takes for the physical traces of nicotine to leave your system; in fact most of it leaves within 24 hours, and any withdrawal pangs are so slight you'll barely be aware of them – even if you've been vaping huge, frequent quantities of nicotine.

SO WHY HAS IT BEEN SO HARD TO QUIT UNTIL NOW?

Many vapers have tried to quit with willpower alone or willpower combined with nicotine patches or gum. Yet they have found that they still craved a vape weeks, months, even years after the Little Monster had died. They have applied all their willpower to resist the cravings, but it only takes one offer of a vape at a party, or in some stressful situation, or something as simple as a bust-up with their partner, and the trap door opens up and drags them in once again.

The fact is, if quitting was as straightforward as stopping vaping and waiting for the Little Monster to die, everybody would do it without fail. But there is a second monster, as I've mentioned already –

the Big Monster which lives in the mind – and it's this that keeps nicotine addicts craving it long after they've quit.

The Big Monster is your perception of vaping as a pleasure or crutch. It is created by all the brainwashing from the tobacco industry and companies like JUUL and a whole host of e-cigarette brands. Not only that, but stars of pop, rock, rap and R&B have been paid to promote vaping, along with social media influencers and other role models. And there are even some anti-smoking campaigners who suggest that former smokers who used vaping to quit smoking and now wish to quit vaping should continue vaping rather than attempt to quit and risk a return to smoking.

Some well-meaning but ill-informed folk also perpetuate the myth that nicotine use is a habit, a pleasure, a crutch; that vapers vape because they choose to; that vapers enjoy vaping; and – the greatest myth of all – that vaping and nicotine addiction is hard to stop.

When the Little Monster starts craving nicotine, the minute physical feeling is enough to awake the Big Monster. Without the influence of the Big Monster, it would be easy to dismiss the cries of the Little Monster and carry on with your life without vaping, but the Big Monster interprets that faint, empty feeling as 'I want a vape' and convinces you that the only way to relieve the craving is to vape.

This is the ingenuity of the nicotine trap. Each dose of nicotine causes the craving for the next. And the belief that vaping gives you pleasure or a crutch is reinforced by the feeling of relief as one vape fills the emptiness left behind by the previous one.

YOUR OBJECTIVE

By now you should be beginning to understand why it's so important to prepare your mindset before we move on to the next stages of helping you to quit nicotine. Your mind is currently occupied by a Big Monster which keeps convincing you that the drug is the solution to all your insecurities and discomforts. You believe it because every time you vape you feel a sense of relief and interpret this as pleasure. But the 'pleasure' is nothing more than the partial relief of the mild discomfort caused by the withdrawal symptoms that followed the previous vape. In other words:

THE ONLY PLEASURE FROM VAPING IS THE PARTIAL RELIEF OF THE DISCOMFORT CAUSED BY VAPING

That point is worth repeating.

THE ONLY PLEASURE FROM VAPING IS THE PARTIAL RELIEF OF THE DISCOMFORT CAUSED BY VAPING

It's like wearing tight shoes all day just for the relief of taking them off. Why subject yourself to the pain in the first place?

When a nicotine addict begins to understand how the nicotine trap works, you can see a light click on in their eyes. It's a revelation. Most vapers go through life not even aware that they're in a trap. They think they vape because they choose to (although they can't understand why), or because it helps them to relax (even though it actually makes them more stressed), or helps them to concentrate (even though it's a constant distraction).

Until the nicotine trap is explained, vapers are left with a headful of contradictions that tug them in opposite directions: the tug-of-war of fear. 'I know it's harming me' versus 'how can I go through life without it?' The solution is easy:

KILL THE BIG MONSTER

In order to do that, we need to unravel all the brainwashing that gave birth to the Big Monster in the first place.

ESCAPE IS EASY

A JUULer, IQOSer or e-cigarette user is like a fly in a pitcher plant, but there is one crucial difference. By the time the fly realises it's in danger, the opportunity for escape has passed. The nicotine addict, on the other hand, can escape at any time. The ingenuity of the nicotine trap is also its weakness. You have the power to escape any time you choose because…

YOU ARE YOUR OWN JAILER

Nobody is holding a gun to your head and forcing you to vape. Addiction is what keeps you trapped. Once you've realised this simple fact, you can cure the addiction and walk free any time you want.

Here's a prediction. When you finish this book you will be a happy non-vaper. You will have walked out of the nicotine trap and you will have found the process incredibly easy. Perhaps you find that hard to believe right now.

That's OK. You're not going to be required to do anything hard. In fact, I'm going to make life as easy for you as possible by setting out some simple instructions.

All you have to do is follow the instructions and you can't fail to quit nicotine easily, painlessly and permanently.

A REMINDER OF THE FIRST INSTRUCTION:
FOLLOW ALL THE INSTRUCTIONS

A few hours devoted to reading this book is no time to spend on something as life-changing as quitting nicotine, yet you may well be feeling impatient. Perhaps you're champing at the bit already, wanting to get on with it, or perhaps it's the complete reverse – you're thinking about bailing out on the idea because it all seems too good to be true.

If you're in the former category, keep your discipline; don't be tempted to skip ahead and miss out parts of the book. If you're in the latter group, understand one thing: nothing bad is going to happen while you read this book, or afterwards. You're either going to find it easy to stop or not. If you fail, you'll be no worse off than you are now. You really have nothing to lose, so if for no reason other than curiosity, or even simply to prove me wrong, just carry on reading while you carry on vaping or using nicotine in whatever way you use it, and follow the instructions.

We need to make sure that all the brainwashing is unravelled and that the Big Monster is well and truly dead when you come to have your final vape. We can only achieve that if you follow all the instructions. It's like the combination to unlock a safe. I could give you all the numbers for the combination, but if you left any out or didn't put them in the right order, the safe would remain tight shut.

Chapter 4

THE MYTH

IN THIS CHAPTER
• *WE'VE ALL BEEN BRAINWASHED* • *THE ILLUSION OF ENJOYMENT*
• *YOUR SURVIVAL TOOLKIT* • *WHO'S GIVING THE ORDERS?*
• *DISTINGUISHING INSTINCT FROM INTELLECT* • *CHANGE YOUR PERCEPTION*

You should now understand that the real reason you vape is purely to satisfy the Little Monster which you created when you had your first dose of nicotine, and the only reason you believe that vaping will relieve your craving is because of a Big Monster in your mind which interprets the cries of the Little Monster as 'I want a vape.' The next step is to recognise that you have been brainwashed.

WE'VE ALL BEEN BRAINWASHED

Nicotine addicts and non-nicotine addicts are brainwashed into believing a myth. The brainwashing is relentless and all of us are exposed to it from the day we are born. It comes in many forms and from many sources and you rarely hear it challenged. The net result of all the brainwashing is the myth that nicotine offers some sort of pleasure or crutch.

The brainwashing is so all-consuming that even non-nicotine addicts believe it. Most people who have never smoked or vaped, or been inclined to smoke or vape, will believe there may be something relaxing or stress-relieving in nicotine. You can't really blame them; their attitude is often one of incredulity: 'There's no way that smokers or vapers would suffer all the dangers and disadvantages of what they do if they didn't get something from it.'

Even nicotine addicts who appear to do it for pure pleasure give away their true feelings. I'm talking about those who only smoke or vape occasionally. The implication is that they are in control, choosing where and when they do it, unlike those who constantly tug on their device throughout the day.

But those casual vapers are caught in exactly the same trap and they know it. They love to tell you that they can go days without doing it if they have to. Now why would they do that if they thought vaping was a genuine pleasure or crutch?

A lot of people love exercising. You never hear them bragging about how long they can go without exercising.

They would exercise all the time if they could because they love it and it makes them feel good. For them, exercising is a genuine pleasure. Vapers are always trying to fight the urge to do it. What kind of a pleasure is that?

As long as you continue to perceive vaping or nicotine use as a pleasure or crutch, you will always find it hard to quit. But as soon as you can see that any perception of pleasure or crutch is an illusion created by a combination of brainwashing and addiction, you will find it easy and enjoyable to quit.

THE ILLUSION OF ENJOYMENT

We all know the pitfalls of vaping. The health risks are becoming better known, and increasingly worrying, but rather than putting us off ever trying a vape the negative publicity adds to the myth. The element of danger, the taboo, the rebellion… this is what attracts some youngsters to vaping for the first time. For others it can be the complete reverse. Products like JUUL came on to the market with a terrific marketing fanfare, sleek advertising and the cynical targeting of youngsters. The products were designed to look stylish, modern and cool. It never occurred to the youngsters lured into trying out JUUL that by doing so they were risking a lifetime of addiction or any lasting physical damage.

The bright colours and fresh flavours are all part of the lure, rather like the nectar in the pitcher plant – but they're not the reason we continue to vape. It has nothing to do with how the vape tastes or smells – it's simply down to the addiction.

Often vapers dismiss it as just a habit they got into. This betrays the shame and helplessness they feel. They know there's nothing good about vaping, nothing to be proud of. It's become a drain on their finances and they're increasingly aware of the potential impact on their health and relationships, yet they've also found themselves powerless to stop doing it. Whenever they summon up the willpower to attempt to quit, they feel deprived and miserable and return to vaping.

If the fly could see it was in a trap before it started to slide down the pitcher plant, it would fly away. You have that chance. Take it!

The excuses for vaping keep changing, but the real reason never does. Despite reaching the stage where it's obvious that it's giving you no pleasure or crutch, you keep doing it to try and end the empty, insecure feeling that the first shot of the drug created. But each dose does not end that feeling, it does the very opposite.

EACH SHOT OF NICOTINE REKINDLES THE CRAVING AND ENSURES THAT YOU SUFFER IT OVER AND OVER FOR THE REST OF YOUR LIFE

The only way to stop the craving is to stop feeding the Little Monster. Very soon it will die and the mild physical discomfort will stop. There are two ways to kill the Little Monster: the hard way or Easyway. Kill the Big Monster first and quitting is easy.

YOUR SURVIVAL TOOLKIT

Think back to that first ever vape you had. All your instincts will have been telling you to avoid it, yet something in your mind made you persevere. If you had listened to your instincts, you would not be in this predicament now.

The human body is an incredible machine. Its powers of recovery are extraordinary. We abuse our bodies with all sorts of poisons – nicotine, alcohol, sugar, etc. – yet our bodies keep soldiering on. Any time you decide to stop abusing yourself and lead a healthier lifestyle, your body recovers with extraordinary speed. It's not just your body that feels healthier either. Your mind responds to the way you live too. Eat healthily and take exercise, and you feel better mentally as well as physically. The reverse is also true: abuse your body and your mental health suffers too.

You have been equipped with a remarkable natural toolkit for survival. It consists of a number of reflexes, such as fear, pain, fatigue, etc., which all serve to help keep you alive. Ironically, we tend to regard these things as weaknesses. Without them, we would not last very long.

For example, we tend to equate fear with cowardice, but without fear you would wander blindly into deadly dangers, such as fire, heights and water. Fear is an instinct designed to help us avoid danger. When threatened, our fear sends us into survival mode: fight, flight or freeze. Without it, our ancestors wouldn't have survived.

Vapers often complain that they suffer with nerves and need to vape to calm themselves. Beside the fact that vaping will only make their nervous state worse, they're overlooking the fact that nerves are part of the survival toolkit. If you jump out of your skin every time a door slams, that's the same instinctive response as the one that sends the birds flying from the trees at the sound of a gunshot. OK, so you may feel you overreact to sudden noises, but it's an important part of our survival instinct. When you've quit nicotine, you will find your nerves are a lot less frayed.

Fatigue and pain are other instincts we try to fight off with caffeine drinks and painkillers. We ignore the warning signs. Fatigue is your body's way of telling you that you need rest. Pain is your body's way of telling you it's being attacked and you need to tackle the cause and not keep trying to suppress the symptoms with drugs.

By tackling the symptoms rather than the cause, as so much of modern medicine does, we don't just allow the cause to continue – meaning the pain will get steadily worse – we also develop a tolerance against the drugs. That means we need bigger and bigger doses to get the same effect. It's the same downward spiral that occurs with any drug, including nicotine.

Your senses are a vital part of your survival toolkit and when you had your first ever vape your senses of taste and smell would have questioned what you were doing. The smell and the flavour might have been based on natural substances – but the strange, synthetic undernote or aftertaste would have crossed your mind and made you question your actions.

We share these survival tools with the rest of the animal kingdom, yet while all other animals heed the warnings, we choose to override them. Why do you think that is?

WHO'S GIVING THE ORDERS?

The tool that distinguishes human beings from the rest of the animal kingdom is intellect. It is another wonderful tool. Our intellect enables us to make judgements based not only on what is happening in the here and now, but also on past experiences and even the experiences of others. It also helps us to predict future outcomes by using our imagination and projecting that experience on to hypothetical situations.

Thanks to this incredible tool, we have created sophisticated civilisations with remarkable architecture, art, literature, music, philosophy, sport and science. We no longer need to hunt for food, gather our own fuel for warmth or fight off predators. We have been able to share our intellect with future generations, ensuring the constant progression of technology and ideas.

But our intellect has also led us into disaster. Wars, weapons, drugs, slavery, prejudice and murder are all products of human intellect. But this hasn't dampened our pride in our intellect, nor our faith in the power of human reason. And so, when our intellect and our instincts conflict, it's our intellect from which we take orders.

The problem begins at birth, when the shock of coming into the world leaves us clinging to our mothers for security. In childhood, our parents comfort us with fairy tales and other examples of make-believe: the tooth fairy, the Easter bunny, Father Christmas...

Then comes the day when we discover that none of this fantasy world exists. Our view of our parents changes. It begins to dawn on us that they are not the towers of strength we thought they were; they're fallible, and they have weaknesses and fears just like we do.

The disillusionment leaves a void, an empty, insecure feeling, which we instinctively want to fill. We begin to let other people into our lives to fill the void and with them come other influences. We look to people who appear to have the confidence we crave: rock stars, film stars, sports stars, TV celebrities, models. These people become our role models and we copy their behaviour in the hope that it will lead us to be more like them – or the way we perceive them, anyway. If they dye their hair, we dye our hair. If they go to clubs, we go to clubs. If they drink, we drink. If they smoke, we smoke. If they vape, we vape.

Instead of becoming complete, strong, secure and unique individuals in our own right, we become impressionable fans, leaving ourselves wide open to suggestion. But we don't want our insecurities to show; we want to look self-assured, confident, in control, grown-up. So we begin to mimic the mannerisms of other apparently confident individuals. We think they look cool when they smoke or vape and drink and we know smoking, or vaping and drinking are 'grown-up' things to do because that's what we've always been told and that's what we've always observed.

And so we see smoking or vaping as a fast track to adulthood – in fact, more often than not, vaping appears to surpass smoking in its prestige. In the beginning, adults hadn't caught on to it as much as they have today, so it seemed to be a radical, different, modern, twenty-first century pastime for a youngster to engage with, and this is something that was reinforced by vaping advertising and marketing. Everything we have ever been told, including the warnings that continue to come thick and fast, leaves us in no doubt that vaping is a rite of passage.

The desire for security is instinctive. The belief that vaping provides security is intellectual. It's a myth that has been put in your mind by a lifetime of brainwashing. As humans, our incredible ability to communicate and absorb information is matched by our ability to communicate and absorb misinformation.

When you came to vape that first ever time, your instincts did everything in their power to stop you. Or perhaps you had been lured by the messaging of the nicotine pusher corporations – that there was absolutely nothing to fear and everything to gain, and were led, in all innocence, towards something you believed to be entirely benign.

You then become accustomed to the process of inhaling and exhaling the vape cloud and another sophisticated process goes into action: you build a tolerance to the poison. By the time you think you've acquired the knack of vaping and have experimented with flavours and nicotine strengths, you're already well and truly hooked and the cycle of addiction is drawing you deeper and deeper into the trap. All that awaits you is the miserable life of a nicotine addict.

DISTINGUISHING INSTINCT FROM INTELLECT

If you trusted your instincts over your intellect, you would never have inhaled your first vape. Like so many of the human race, you didn't, but it's never too late to learn.

As I pointed out earlier on, most of the time you vape without paying any attention to it whatsoever. You might say it's an instinctive reflex, but it is not a natural instinct designed as part of your survival toolkit. It's a reflex created by brainwashing and addiction. If we do something enough times, the brain is rewired.

So how do we distinguish our natural survival instincts from the unnatural reaction to being brainwashed? It's actually a case of distinguishing fact from fiction.

The brainwashing creates the belief in your mind that vaping offers some kind of pleasure or crutch. The cycle of addiction, whereby each dose of nicotine offers partial relief from the craving created by the one before, convinces you that you do get some pleasure or comfort when you do it. Remember, this is no more of a pleasure than the relief of taking off tight shoes. But, you might ask, if you believe that you're gaining some pleasure from vaping, what does it matter if that perception is based on fact or fiction?

Would you remain grateful to the thief for giving you £10 of the £100 he secretly stole from you once you found out about his ruse? Of course not.

It matters because vaping does the complete opposite of what you believe it does.

VAPING MAKES ALL VAPERS MISERABLE

BUT YOU ONLY REALISE JUST HOW MISERABLE WHEN YOU ESCAPE

If the delusion really made you happy, you might argue that it's worth all the money and the risks to your health. But it doesn't. Vaping makes you irritable, self-despising and frightened. And the more you do it, the worse you feel.

When you satisfy a genuine instinct like hunger or thirst, it gives you genuine pleasure and a lasting feeling of satisfaction and wellbeing. When you vape, all you get is temporary and partial relief, which is quickly replaced by insecurity and emptiness. This void is created by the very thing that you take to relieve it. But you keep taking it because you believe in the myth. The only way to remove this artificial void is to remove the addiction.

Unravelling the brainwashing so you can distinguish genuine instinctive fact from brainwashed intellectual fiction is actually incredibly easy. All you need to do is channel your intellect in the right direction and use it to replace misinformed responses with correctly informed ones.

CHANGE YOUR PERCEPTION

To help you see through the myth, it helps to look at your addiction through the eyes of a non-nicotine addict. You can get an idea of how that might appear by thinking about how you regard a heroin addict. Apart from the tiny proportion of vapers who are also addicted to heroin, vapers have no problem in seeing that heroin will do absolutely nothing for them and that they neither need nor want it. You don't have to keep convincing yourself.

So why do you think heroin addicts have this great desire to inject themselves with the drug? Do you envy them? Or do you thank your lucky stars that you're not going through the same hell as them? If you could help them, wouldn't you tell them to stop? Why do you think they can't see their predicament in the same way as you? Could it be because their perspective has been distorted by the drug?

Now consider this: non-vapers regard you and your predicament in exactly the same way. It's clear to them that there is no pleasure and that vaping leaves you feeling more insecure, less relaxed and distracted. Their perception is not distorted by any drug.

THEY CAN SEE THE FACTS AS CLEARLY AS YOU CAN SEE THE PLIGHT OF THE HEROIN ADDICT

If you're still clinging to the myth that vaping offers you some sort of pleasure or crutch, it's time to change your perception. You should already be seeing your addiction in a new light. It's not enough, though, just to understand the logic in what I've told you so far.

YOU HAVE TO ACCEPT IT

That means questioning everything that you believe to be true about vaping, including what I've told you, and examining it carefully until you see the truth. This leads me to remind you of the fifth instruction.

FIFTH INSTRUCTION: KEEP AN OPEN MIND

Perhaps you think you are an open-minded person. But the mind can be easily fooled into believing something that is untrue. Once we believe in something we tend to close our minds to anything that contradicts that belief. The nicotine trap relies on this aspect of human intellect. Only when you question your belief with an open mind can you determine fact from fiction.

VAPING DOES NOTHING FOR YOU WHATSOEVER

Chapter 5

FIRST STEPS TO FREEDOM

IN THIS CHAPTER
•NO MORE STOPPING AND STARTING •HARD DRUGS
•FEAR OF SUCCESS •A POSITIVE APPROACH

You may be wondering how you can undo a lifetime's brainwashing just by reading this book. Don't worry, we normally succeed in around five hours at our live seminars. Like anything that is not built on solid foundations, the brainwashing is as fragile as a house of cards and will collapse in an instant. All you have to do is give it a shake.

NO MORE STOPPING AND STARTING

Changing your mindset is all it takes to remove the desire to vape. We now have a simple set of tasks.

- identify what's wrong with your current mindset

- remove that from your way of thinking

- let logic and reason undo the brainwashing.

Logic and reasoning are your dynamite. When you apply them to your reasons for vaping, the whole argument collapses and you are left with no lingering desire to vape. The problem for vapers is that they don't apply logic and reason because the addiction distorts their sense of reality.

This method shows you how to apply logic and reason. It's as simple as that. Easyway shows you how to light the fuse to bring the brainwashing collapsing down.

Our objective is to help you quit PERMANENTLY. How many times have you vowed that you're going to quit vaping, only to fall into the trap again?

Vapers are notorious for repeatedly stopping and starting. To the non-nicotine addict, this is illogical. If you like doing it, why keep trying to quit? If you don't like doing it, why keep starting again?

Falling back into the trap is not like falling into a physical trap. If you fell into a pit of stagnant water, you would make sure you didn't go anywhere near that pit again, wouldn't you? But the nicotine trap is not a physical trap; it's a mental trap, based on illusion.

Vapers who stop and start again have not seen through the illusion.

All vapers wish they could quit. That's why they're always trying to do so. As well as all the logical reasons for quitting – the health risks, the cost, the smell, etc. – you know vaping doesn't make you happy. On the contrary, it makes you feel like a miserable slave.

Yet despite this, the vapers who stop and start again never remove the desire for vaping. They haven't seen through the myth. They're still being fooled by the illusion. It's as illogical as thinking there's a good reason for falling into a pit of stagnant water, but addiction overrides logic.

Do you want to be a non-nicotine addict? Then you need to understand the one real difference between nicotine addicts and non-nicotine addicts. It's not that non-addicts have been spared the brainwashing – they haven't. Neither is it that they had the willpower to resist getting hooked – you don't need willpower to be a non-addict. Nor that they are wired differently – it has nothing to do with genetics. The real difference is that non-addicts never have the desire to vape.

Anyone who retains a desire to vape will feel deprived if they can't do it. They will need willpower to fight the feeling of deprivation and they will be forever vulnerable to falling back into the trap when their willpower runs out.

Remove your desire to vape and you will become a happy non-vaper

EASILY, IMMEDIATELY AND PAINLESSLY

And you won't need willpower.

People who have never been addicted to nicotine don't have the desire to vape though they may still be tempted to try it. They have been subjected to all the brainwashing and they may believe that there must be some pleasure or crutch in vaping, but they have been able to make a logical choice not to subject themselves to a life of nicotine addiction. That is because their mind is not controlled by nicotine addiction. The exception to this may be those unfortunate souls fooled into thinking that vaping is a zero risk, non-addictive, enjoyable, benign, experience akin to eating a bag of sweets.

People who become happy non-vapers with Easyway also have no desire to vape. They have an advantage over people who have never vaped because they *know* there is no pleasure or crutch to be gained from doing it and they have not had to use reason to outweigh temptation.

EASYWAY REMOVES THE TEMPTATION
TO VAPE ALTOGETHER

When you know for a fact that vaping does absolutely nothing for you whatsoever, any desire disappears. See through the myth and it becomes easy to avoid falling into the trap again. Once you're free, you'll be more likely to start believing in Father Christmas again than fall back into the trap. All you need to do is follow the instructions.

HARD DRUGS

We regard heroin as a hard drug and nicotine as a social drug. I'm not suggesting you start taking heroin and, even if I did, I doubt you would pay any attention. More likely you would put this book down and write me off as mad.

Instead, we're talking about another drug that is very dangerous. People make a fortune from selling it and deliberately try to get their customers hooked so they have a steadily increasing income. It's highly addictive and if you try it you're likely to get hooked straight away, and remain hooked for the rest of your life.

It's also very expensive but whatever the cost addicts always make sure they find the money, regardless of what other sacrifices they have to make.

When you take the drug, you become increasingly lethargic and your immune system weakens, leaving you susceptible to all sorts of diseases. Worst of all, it destroys your nervous system by stealth, as well as your courage, your confidence and your ability to concentrate. It makes you despise yourself for being a slave to something you detest, but the more it drags you down the more you depend on it.

And what does this drug do for you?

ABSOLUTELY NOTHING

NOT ONE SINGLE THING

As no doubt you've surmised, I'm not talking about heroin; I'm talking about nicotine. If I tried to sell you a drug using the description above, would you buy it? Or would you throw me out, just like you would if I tried to persuade you to take heroin? After all, who in their right mind would cough up such a fortune to put themselves through all that misery?

We have no difficulty in seeing heroin addiction as a vile, pitiful, deadly condition, yet we have a distorted view of vaping. We need to make sure you can see your addiction exactly as you see the heroin addict's addiction. To do this, you need to disregard the images portrayed in society. It's easy to associate heroin with addiction, slavery, poverty, misery, squalor and death because you haven't been bombarded with images of happy, laughing heroin addicts. Vapers, on the other hand, are portrayed as cool, in control, stylish, beautiful people. The inference is that these vapers are happy because they are vaping.

It's essential that you see through this illusion. You don't just need to tell yourself it's untrue; you *know* it's untrue because you know how vaping makes you feel. Disregard the popular image of vapers, the one that is promoted by million-dollar advertising campaigns designed to lure you and your kids into a lifetime's addiction, and look at your own evidence. Look at the nicotine addicts you know in real life. How many of them live up to the imagery? Remember, beautiful, stylish, cool people aren't made to look beautiful, stylish and cool by vaping – they are already all of those things.

FEAR OF SUCCESS

We'll soon begin the process of stripping away the illusions that have kept you in the nicotine trap. Our goal is the removal of all your doubts about wanting to quit. Those doubts are fuelled by the chief ally of addiction:

FEAR

Vapers are held back from trying to quit by numerous fears:

- **fear of being unable to enjoy meals, drinks or social occasions**

- **fear of being unable to handle stress**

- **fear of being unable to concentrate**

- **fear of having to go through some terrible trauma to get free**

- **fear of having to resist temptation for the rest of their life.**

They fear that they won't have the resilience to cope with these challenges and so any attempt to quit will end in dismal failure. What they're really afraid of is success.

The fear of failure is a spur. It drives actors to learn their lines, athletes to practise their skills, pilots to check their instruments, etc., etc. There is no logic in not trying to quit because you're afraid of failure. The calamity you're afraid of has already happened.

YOU ARE A VAPER!

By not trying to quit, you guarantee that the unthinkable happens. You remain a vaper. Instead, think about everything you stand to gain. How proud will your family and friends be? More importantly, how proud will *you* feel?

The fears listed above amount to the fear of success. 'If I quit, life will be tough.' Nicotine addicts have been fooled into thinking it provides them with a crutch in stressful situations and that there will be no pleasure in life without it. The thought of never vaping again is frightening.

Non-vapers manage to enjoy life and cope with stressful situations with ease. In fact, they cope better and enjoy life more. The only reason you might think life will be worse without nicotine is because your addiction makes you miserable when you don't vape. As long as you continue to feed the Little Monster, this will be the case. Rid your life of nicotine and the fear goes too.

You are only part of the way into Easyway and you may be finding it hard to imagine just how good life will be without vaping. Believe me, you will soon be looking back on this moment thinking: 'I can't believe I feel this good.'

Not only will you feel healthier and more energetic but you will also notice a marked improvement in your confidence, courage and concentration too.

A POSITIVE APPROACH

So far, we have concentrated on preparing your mindset to unravel the brainwashing and strip away the illusions that have kept you trapped. There are two more instructions I want to remind you about as you look forward to making your escape. First of all, I will now repeat the third instruction.

THIRD INSTRUCTION: START OFF IN A HAPPY FRAME OF MIND

If you have been wrestling with the fear of success, there will be concerns in your mind about what you are about to achieve. Vapers who think they are going to be required to make a sacrifice will approach the attempt to quit with a sense of doom and gloom. There is no reason to feel miserable.

YOU ARE NOT GIVING UP ANYTHING

Instead you are making wonderful gains. Every nicotine addict dreams of waking up in the morning with the sense of freedom you will feel when you reach the end of this book. Allow yourself to imagine how good life is going to be and get excited about what you are about to achieve. This is a fantastic moment in your life. And I'll now remind you about the fourth instruction.

FOURTH INSTRUCTION: THINK POSITIVELY

That means:

BEGIN, NOT WITH A FEELING OF DOOM AND GLOOM, BUT INSTEAD WITH A FEELING OF ELATION AND EXCITEMENT

Remember, if you follow all of the instructions, nothing can stop you from escaping. Let go of the fear and get free.

We've established the real reasons you vape. You are now armed with the knowledge that when you started JUULing or using IQOS or e-cigarettes, or using other nicotine products, you were dragged into a trap: nicotine addiction. This trap distorts logic and tricks its victims into believing that relief from their restlessness lies in the very thing that's causing it: nicotine. You should now understand that the really unpleasant and noticeable physical feelings you've felt in the past when you attempted to quit were not caused by nicotine withdrawal, but were the physical reaction to a mental process which is in itself triggered by the extremely mild physical withdrawal of nicotine.

The Little Monster (the physical withdrawal) is a virtually imperceptible feeling, so slight most vapers aren't even aware of it while they sleep. This very slight physical feeling (the Little Monster) pokes the Big Monster (the brainwashing and the mental process), which creates unpleasant physical feelings.

It works like this:

SLIGHT PHYSICAL WITHDRAWAL

MENTAL PROCESS: 'I WANT A VAPE BUT CAN'T HAVE ONE.'

PHYSICAL UNPLEASANTNESS: 'AGGGH'

Our next task is to begin the process of releasing you from the nicotine trap by dismantling the myth that vaping provides some sort of pleasure or crutch. It is this myth that creates the desire to vape. Remove that desire and escape from the trap is easy.

The myth is reinforced by a number of other myths that are put out there as facts by tobacco companies and companies like JUUL and sometimes even by organisations attempting to help nicotine addicts. With your mind corrupted by these myths, it's no wonder you have been unable to quit vaping up until now.

We are going to tackle seven of these myths:

- that vaping helps you relax

- that you can't quit without willpower

- that quitting requires you to make a sacrifice

- that you might have an addictive personality

- that vaping helps you concentrate

- that vaping helps with weight control and appetite suppression

- that vaping reduces depression or is an expression of self-harm.

By the time we've finished dismantling these myths, you will be feeling much more confident about your ability to quit easily, painlessly and permanently. That's a very exciting feeling. You can begin to imagine life without JUUL, IQOS or any form of nicotine; you'll be healthier, more energetic, better off, free.

So let's get started. Remember to follow all the instructions. Keep an open mind, make no assumptions and question everything. The truth will become obvious. And remember to carry on vaping while you progress through the book, without changing the level of nicotine you use in your device. I don't want you to waste any time or brainpower wondering whether you should or shouldn't do so. Just carry on as you are until you're ready to have your final vape. I'll guide you through that amazing ritual when the time comes. And please don't worry if the prospect makes you nervous or anxious – that's perfectly understandable. This book is exactly the length it needs to be... if we could achieve the result in fewer words, we'd do so. So stick with it, regardless of how positive or negative you feel; you have absolutely nothing to lose and everything to gain.

Chapter 6

THE ILLUSION OF PLEASURE

IN THIS CHAPTER

- *PLEASURE OR CRUTCH?* • *I ENJOY THE SMELL AND TASTE*
- *MY SPECIAL VAPES* • *VAPING EASES MY STRESS*
- *LET GO OF UNNECESSARY STRESS* • *IT'S JUST A HABIT*
- *EASYWAY REMOVES TEMPTATION*

---

*As long as you stick with the belief that vaping gives you some
sort of pleasure or crutch, you will not be able to free yourself from
the nicotine trap. It's essential, then, for me to make sure you fully
understand that any pleasure you think you get from nicotine is a
complete illusion.*

I'm going to make a powerful statement:

YOU HAVEN'T ENJOYED A SINGLE JUUL, IQOS OR E-CIGARETTE YOU'VE EVER HAD

Now don't get me wrong – there's no doubt that you've 'enjoyed'
tremendous 'relief' when vaping after a long period of time without
being allowed to; after a long flight, train journey or an attempt to
quit. Yet that feeling of enjoyment and relief is nothing more than the
feeling you'd get if you wore shoes that were a size too small all day. It

would feel fabulous when you took them off. But would you do that? Of course not! We go out of our way to select our shoes carefully – so they fit just right.

You owe nicotine absolutely nothing. No more than you'd be grateful to the thief who stole £100 from you and 'gifted' you £10… once you discovered the con, you'd never be grateful to the thief again.

PLEASURE OR CRUTCH?

It is widely assumed, by vapers and non-vapers alike, that the effect of vaping must deliver something positive – otherwise why would people keep doing it?

We all know that there are inherent dangers in vaping – more and more are being disclosed to us on a virtually monthly basis – so the assumption is that there must be something pretty special about it to make vapers disregard all these negatives and carry on spending vast amounts of money on nicotine.

The perceived pleasure of vaping seems to enhance social occasions, make drinks more enjoyable, round off a meal or just put the finishing touch to a relaxing, satisfying moment. The perceived crutch lies in nicotine's apparent ability to help you relax, take your mind off the stresses of life and concentrate.

In fact, all of these perceived pleasures and crutches are illusory. JUUL, IQOS, e-cigarettes, snus, dip, nicotine gum and in fact any nicotine product actually do nothing of the sort.

On the contrary, they are antisocial; they can interfere with the taste of meals and drinks; they make a relaxing situation feel edgy; they add to your stress and they destroy your concentration. You only have to observe how embarrassed most vapers are when using their devices. It only becomes less embarrassing when they are in the company of other addicts. That's why smokers and vapers seem to have that camaraderie at parties. It's a case of: 'Thank goodness – I'm not the only one here!'

But let's examine the claim that vaping can help you take your mind off things at times of stress and help you concentrate at a time when you're required to focus. Think about it: how can the same drug take your mind off things and help you concentrate at the same time?

The same person who claims that vaping distracts their mind in a stressful situation will, in the next breath, also claim that it provides no distraction whatsoever when it comes to concentration – in fact they claim it helps them to do so. If you haven't immediately grasped the contradictory nature of those two claims, then please consider carefully what I just said before moving on.

YOU'RE STRESSED AND WANT TO BE DISTRACTED FROM YOUR PROBLEMS – SO YOU VAPE

YOU NEED TO FOCUS AND CONCENTRATE WITHOUT DISTRACTIONS – SO YOU VAPE

Can you see how one justification is the complete opposite of the other?

There is no genuine pleasure or crutch to be derived from vaping; we only think there is because of the brainwashing and the way the nicotine trap twists our perception.

The fact is, our addiction to nicotine makes us incapable of doing anything without a vape before, during or after a stressful or focus-requiring event. It's like the neighbour's burglar alarm which goes off for hours, and the feeling of relief when it finally stops. That is the only reason you believe that nicotine helps you to focus (you are removing the aggravation of wanting a vape) and the only reason you believe it helps you cope with stress (you constantly have the aggravation of wanting a vape and if you can't have one it actually adds to your stress levels).

Am I really expecting you to believe that nobody ever enjoyed a single vape? It seems too far-fetched. How could anyone create an illusion on such a massive scale?

It's all to do with every vaper's reluctance to admit to their misery. Instead of admitting to being a helpless slave, they choose to perpetuate the myth that vaping gives them some kind of pleasure or crutch. There is no need for putting a brave face on it. You're in it together with all the other nicotine addicts on the planet, but you can admit the truth here:

VAPING DOES NOTHING FOR YOU WHATSOEVER

Although I expect you're beginning to understand exactly what I mean, please don't worry if you require further evidence. Every doubt, every question on your mind at this point will be covered before I ask you to have your final dose of nicotine. So let's examine those illusions and make sure we can see through them.

I ENJOY THE SMELL AND TASTE

Some people say they like the smell of their vape. There is no doubt that the industry has worked extremely hard to produce exciting and tempting flavours and smells with which to snare people. Yet in most cases, after the initial moment, the smell becomes quite unpleasant to some – not just to the person vaping but to those around them. But even if you love the smell of your vape, is that reason enough to poison yourself and risk remaining a slave to nicotine and doing yourself harm? I like the smell of roses, but I could easily live without it. If my life depended on never smelling another rose again, I would have absolutely no problem with going along with that. I'm sure you feel the same. And, of course, some vaping ingredients and devices barely smell at all. We don't vape for the smell or the taste – although no doubt we think we do.

When a vaper quits with the willpower method and is desperately trying to resist the temptation to do it, the smell of a vape cloud might be enough to make them crack, but that's not because they adore the smell of vape more than life itself. It's because they associate the smell with the relief of the craving for nicotine.

Don't become obsessed with the idea that you like the smell of vape. It probably sounds weird, but I like the smell of petrol. I don't hang around petrol stations or carry a small bottle of petrol on me to sniff it every now and then, though. It doesn't matter if you like the smell; all that matters is that you get rid of the belief that you vape because you like the smell. That's not why you vape. You vape in spite of the smell rather than because of it.

Although you might believe that you love the smell of your butter-scotch, bubble gum, candy floss or gummy bear 'vape juice', I can assure you that no one is following you around attempting to inhale it themselves. The smell in this case isn't from a relatively benign source such as a sweet shop (who doesn't love the smell that blows out of those?): in the case of a vape cloud its source is truly revolting. From the vape device, via the vaper's mouth, trachea and lungs and straight back out into the poor passer-by's face.

One of the therapists at our London centre came up with an excellent analogy. He asserted that it's more likely that someone would eat a 'camel dung sandwich' if it smelt like bananas or strawberries and cream, but essentially it doesn't change the fact that it's a camel dung sandwich. And as soon as someone is made aware of that fact, no one, not even someone on one of those weird TV programmes where participants are set repulsive eating challenges, would actually eat it.

MOST VAPES OCCUR WITHOUT THE VAPER PAYING ANY ATTENTION AT ALL TO THE TASTE OR SMELL

No one vapes because they enjoy the taste or smell; they only think they do because they associate the taste and smell with the illusion of relief and the illusion of pleasure that they suffer as a nicotine addict.

MY SPECIAL VAPES

One of the strongest illusions vapers suffer is that there are certain relaxed occasions when a vape seems particularly special. Typical occasions are first thing in the morning, after a meal, with a drink, during a break at work, when you first get home, after exercise and after love-making.

These are all classic occasions when vapers are eager to mark the moment by sucking poison into their lungs. All of these occasions have one thing in common: they follow a period of abstinence. The Little Monster has been kept waiting longer than usual, so it is constantly prodding the Big Monster, and so the feeling of relief once the vaper is able to finally vape seems greater as a consequence.

The first thing in the morning vape is a strange one. It seems special because you've gone without nicotine for hours. So strong is the human body that it has started to recover overnight, so it is more sensitive to the poison. Vapers talk about the hit they get from that first vape of the day. This is actually their body recoiling from the poison.

Other vapers talk about the 'buzz' or 'high' from vaping. Wake up! That isn't a buzz or a high – it's just a dizzy sensation caused by the poisoning effect of the nicotine. If you had the same feeling after eating an oyster, you'd start to panic. Most vapers find even that wears off after a week or two, because the body builds a tolerance to the poison.

You can get exactly the same feeling by holding your breath for longer than is comfortable or from spinning around in a circle for 20 seconds. Calling it a buzz or a high is just something we do in a vain attempt to justify our vaping. If you've ever experienced one of life's *REAL* highs, you'll know that the notion of a high caused by nicotine is a nonsense.

Going back to those special occasions, ask yourself this: would those moments cease to be special if you took away the vape?

How does a non-vaper feel after a meal?

THEY FEEL GREAT!

How does a vaper feel if they're unable to vape at that time?

LOUSY

They hit the fire button and how do they feel?

GREAT!

(IN OTHER WORDS, THEY FEEL THE SAME AS A NON-VAPER FEELS!)

GET IT?

How does a non-vaper feel when they hook up with some friends in a bar or coffee shop?

GREAT!

How does a vaper feel in that same situation if they're unable to vape?

LOUSY!

How do they feel when they're able to take their fix of nicotine?

GREAT!

(AT THAT POINT THEY FEEL LIKE A NON-NICOTINE ADDICT FEELS ALL THE TIME)

I'll keep going for a little longer. By now I hope you understand exactly what I'm saying, but let's make sure.

How does a non-vaper feel after sex?

FABULOUS!

How does a vaper feel at this point if they're unable to vape?

LOUSY!

(THEY THEN FIRE UP THEIR VAPE AND FEEL FABULOUS... LIKE A NON-VAPER FEELS)

Actually, this example differs slightly in that often a vaper will tend to 'get love-making over with' as a matter of urgency – just as soon as the thought of vaping enters their mind. Meanwhile, while the vaper's puffing away on their post-coital vape, the happy non-vaper is happily carrying on making love, or enjoying doing it all over again, or simply lying wrapped in their lover's arms. You can see why sometimes having a partner who vapes can be very frustrating and unrewarding for a non-vaper.

Incidentally, if your partner vapes and has no intention of quitting, or fails to quit at the same time as you, please don't worry. Other than the issue mentioned above, which I'm sure love will conquer, it won't cause you a problem.

In the past, if they've carried on vaping when you attempted to quit, it might have made you envious or caused temptation because nicotine was always around the house. But this time you're going to be truly free, not remotely tempted to vape, so it really won't bother you if your partner, friends or colleagues continue.

More about special vapes, like the one during a break from work: well... there's no doubt that there is great camaraderie among vapers and smokers in the smoking shelter at work. So after you've quit, make sure you carry on taking those breaks. Go for a 'no-vape-break'. You don't want to miss out on the chat and the gossip and the friendship of those breaks just because you've quit vaping. The great thing about being a happy non-vaper is that you can choose when to take your breaks, rather than be compelled to by the Little Monster and the Big Monster. If it's pouring down with rain or freezing cold, you can give it a miss. You can pick and choose when and where to take a break. Other than the phoney relief of the addiction, it's the break that the vaper enjoys – not the vape.

When you quit vaping you will discover that all of these scenarios are not only special regardless of the vape; they are actually more special without it.

As a vaper, you're never fully relaxed. Therefore, vaping actually spoils relaxing situations by adding an unnecessary layer of stress. Which brings us to the next popular myth.

VAPING EASES MY STRESS

How can something that creates stress ease stress?

Whenever you vape you feed the Little Monster and thus give yourself some temporary relief from the craving. When you don't understand the nature of the trap you're in, you interpret this relief as a genuine easing of your stress level. Before the vape you feel stressed; as you vape you feel less stressed. And so you jump to the simple and obvious conclusion.

Stress is a fact of life, suffered by vapers and non-vapers alike. But nicotine addicts suffer an additional layer of stress caused by nicotine withdrawal (the Little Monster) which triggers the even worse feeling of stress (the Big Monster: 'I want a vape – I can't have one – AGGH!'). When you vape, you partially relieve this additional layer of stress. But vaping makes no impact on genuine stress. The truth is it adds to it.

I can guarantee that...

YOU WILL BE LESS STRESSED AS A NON-VAPER

The additional layer of stress is responsible for every vaper's descent into the nicotine trap. Like the fly in the pitcher plant, once you're in the nicotine trap there is only one way to go: down.

UNLESS, OF COURSE, YOU CHOOSE TO ESCAPE

The natural tendency with any addictive drug is to take more, not less. This is because of your body's incredible ability to build a tolerance to the poison. Because of this tolerance, each shot of nicotine can give only partial relief from the nicotine craving. You become increasingly desensitised to the poison, so it takes more of the drug to get the same effect. You gradually and increasingly inhale deeper and more frequently, reduce the gap between vapes and manipulate the nicotine strength as a result

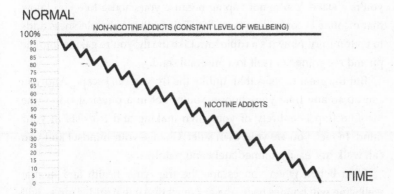

This graph illustrates the nicotine addict's descent as time goes by. Let's say that your level of stress was 'normal' before you started vaping.

This is indicated as 100 per cent on the diagram. As you experience withdrawal from that first vape, you feel a low. You dip down below 100 per cent. Your next vape relieves this feeling but not completely, because of your tolerance to the poison. You certainly couldn't call it a high. At best it's partial and temporary relief. So you don't quite make it back to 100 per cent. The next withdrawal causes a low that takes you down further than before. So the pattern continues, taking you down further and further each time you vape.

All the while, those periods of partial relief are fooling you into thinking you're getting some pleasure from vaping. You keep believing the myth. But with each vape you're falling further and further below 'normal', each time setting yourself a new normal lower than the one before. At the back of your mind the health effects concern you – you brush them away but they remain. This creates a double low.

As your descent accelerates, you have to admit to yourself that you're a slave. You're not vaping because you choose to – you know that nicotine is controlling your life. This feeling of helplessness adds to your misery. Now it's a triple low. Like the fly, you're gazing into the pit and resigning yourself to a miserable end.

But the great news is that, unlike the fly, you *can* escape. And you can do so any time you choose. You're not in a physical trap – the nicotine trap is entirely of your own making and it exists in your mind. In fact, you are your own jailer. Change your mindset and you can walk free easily, immediately and painlessly.

Even better, when you escape the trap your health and mental wellbeing will bounce back up very quickly. All that added stress will lift from your shoulders, you will enjoy the feeling of renewed health and vigour, not to mention more money, and you will experience a feeling of elation.

YIPPEE! I'M FREE!

When you're vaping, you have to suppress your instincts and bury your head in the sand. That's the only way you can maintain the illusion of pleasure. You have to block out the concerns you might have about your health, about the money you're wasting, and the slavery. The pretence is very stressful. When you quit, you don't have to go through that any more. The relief is incredible.

LET GO OF UNNECESSARY STRESS

It's the additional layers of stress which make nicotine addicts miserable. The fear of what vaping is doing to you and the misery of being a slave are stresses that non-vapers don't suffer. You don't have to suffer them either, now that you know you're on the way to becoming a happy non-vaper. Just the aggravation of working out when and where you can have your next vape adds significantly to your stress levels. Even sneaking in crafty vapes in places where you know you really shouldn't adds stress. We kid ourselves that it's an exciting, rebellious thing to do – but it isn't. If we stopped for a moment and looked at ourselves as a non-addict might, whether it's while we're hiding in a toilet cubicle on an aeroplane or during a bathroom break in an important meeting, it would make us feel pathetic and wretched – like a junkie.

Next time you think about the effect your vaping is having on you, let the thought pass without allowing it to make you feel anxious. There is no need to worry any more because you are escaping from the trap. Replace your anxiety with a feeling of anticipation or elation. Instead of letting your thoughts about nicotine become a source of stress, think about all the marvellous gains you're about to make and use the thought as a source of joy.

YOU'RE NOT GOING TO BE A SLAVE ANY
MORE. YOU'RE GOING TO BE FREE!

EXERCISE: I ENJOY THE RITUAL

A lot of people are attracted to vaping by the paraphernalia. Whether it's pods or mods, freebase or salts, flavours, Propylene Glycol or Vegetable Glycerin or whatever – we fool ourselves that the equipment and the ingredients and the vaping create a kind of meaningful ritual that has some kind of integrity. It all has a certain style that appeals to young people in need of an identity. A lot of long-term vapers will also tell you that this is what they enjoy about vaping. The inference is that they wouldn't vape if it wasn't for the ritual of putting the whole thing together.

I want you to go through your usual ritual now. Focus on each part of it: go through the entire ritual from selecting the flavour to preparing the device, right up to the point that you would take a puff.

OK, now stop. Put the device down without taking a puff and think.

How do you feel?

Are you satisfied?

I suspect you're not. No one vapes for the ritual. If they did, they would be happy to stop short of taking a puff. Imagine that! You could spare yourself all the harmful part and the cost and still have the enjoyment of the ritual.

But it doesn't work like that, does it? Vapers only enjoy the ritual of vaping because it's a necessary route to getting their fix. Remember, the only reason anyone vapes or uses dip or any other nicotine product is to get the nicotine.

IT'S JUST A HABIT

When nicotine addicts find themselves running out of excuses, they resort to a more resigned explanation as to why they do it. 'It's just a habit.' They're no longer trying to convince themselves or anyone else that they're in control, but there is still the implication that vaping gives them some kind of pleasure or crutch. It's essential to understand that you vape because you're addicted to a drug and

DRUG ADDICTION IS NOT A HABIT

A habit is a repeated behaviour that you do for the familiarity and comfort of repetition. But you don't vape for the comfort of repetition; you vape to get nicotine to relieve the withdrawal pangs from the previous vape and ease the mental aggravation caused by the Big Monster.

If you believe that you vape because you've fallen into the habit, you will find it hard to quit. You will assume that it's just a weakness in your nature that has made you susceptible to the habit. But when you accept that vaping is an addiction and you understand the nature of the nicotine trap, it's easy to follow the instructions to escape.

Get this clear in your mind. The habit of vaping might trigger the thought of having a vape, but that's not why you vape. In the past, when you've attempted to quit, the habit trigger has caused you to mope for a vape, but remember that was when your Big Monster was still alive; you missed vaping and you felt deprived. This time when you quit you won't feel like you're missing out on anything, so if you habitually experience a trigger – getting off a bus for example – it'll be a moment of happiness, a moment when you can remind yourself how lucky you are to be free, rather than a time for concern. I know you'll find that hard to believe at this point, but I'm sure you understand exactly what I'm saying, just on principle. That's all you need to do as we work through this book.

A further problem with seeing vaping as a habit is that it encourages the belief that you can moderate it, so you can have the occasional vape without falling into the trap again. Get it clear in your mind:

THERE IS NO SUCH THING AS 'JUST THE ONCE'

If you vape just the once, what's to stop you vaping again, and again? If you retain the desire for just one puff of vape, you will not escape the trap.

EASYWAY REMOVES TEMPTATION

The belief that you vape out of habit makes vapers feel stupid. One part of your brain is telling you, 'You're a fool. Stop doing it!' and another part is saying, 'I'm helpless to resist the temptation.'

In fact, vapers are not stupid. They are being conned by a fiendish force called addiction. The temptation exists because you have been brainwashed into believing a myth: that vaping gives you some kind of pleasure or crutch. Even when you reach the point where you can no longer convince yourself that you are getting any pleasure or crutch from vaping, the temptation to go on vaping remains. It is driven by fear. 'How will I be able to cope without nicotine?'

What vapers don't realise is that vaping, far from relieving this fear, causes it. Non-vapers don't suffer it. The problem is that it works back to front. It's when you're not vaping that you notice the empty, insecure feeling that vaping causes. When you inhale the vape, the feeling is partially relieved and your brain is fooled into believing that the vape is your friend. This is how vaping creates the illusion of pleasure.

The more it drags you down, the more you believe you need your 'friend' and the more dependent on the drug you feel.

In order to remove the temptation, all you have to do is see through the illusion of pleasure. Recognise that the empty, insecure feeling you experience when you're not vaping is nicotine craving caused by vaping and that the 'pleasure' you feel when you vape is merely the temporary and partial relief of that craving and the pacification of the Big Monster in your mind.

EXERCISE: DEFINE THE PLEASURE

Assuming you've continued to vape as you've been reading this book, have a vape now. Inhale six deep, glorious lungfuls of the filth. Ask yourself what is so pleasant. What are you actually enjoying about it?

Remember, this is the little pleasure or crutch that you thought you couldn't live without. Now is your chance to really identify what that pleasure or crutch amounts to. Hold the vaping device to your mouth. Focus as it hits your lungs and focus on the taste.

Let vape linger in your nostrils or mouth and focus on the smell. Is it pleasant?

You may well feel a sense of relaxation. It's the same as taking off tight shoes.

Would you deliberately wear tight shoes, just for the relief of taking them off?

Chapter 7

BELIEF NOT WILLPOWER

IN THIS CHAPTER
- *THE WRONG METHOD* •*TIGHTENING THE ROPE*
- *HOW WEAK-WILLED ARE YOU?* •*BEWARE OTHER QUITTERS*
- *CROSSING THE LINE THE EASY WAY*

Most people believe that vapers who fail to quit lack the willpower to make the necessary sacrifice. When you quit with Easyway, there is no sacrifice and so you don't need willpower. In fact, the willpower method is more likely to make your addiction worse.

THE WRONG METHOD
So the solution to ending the nicotine craving is simply NOT to vape. That way you break the cycle of addiction, kill the Little Monster and get free. Wait a minute! Isn't that what all vapers do when they try to quit? Why doesn't it work for them? If it's so easy to quit, why do so many people find it incredibly hard?

SIMPLE: THEY'RE USING THE WRONG METHOD

It's not their fault. A fundamental part of the brainwashing is the myth that it's hard to quit. Just about every so-called expert says so, thus adding to every vaper's fear of trying to quit.

'I'M GOING TO HAVE TO GO THROUGH SOME TERRIBLE TRAUMA.'

This brainwashing is so powerful that vapers actually feel suspicious when they're told that Easyway can help them quit easily and without willpower. It goes against everything they've ever been told about nicotine addiction and it sounds too good to be true. Believe me, that is not the case and I will explain why. With Easyway, there is no painful withdrawal period, no traumatic wrestling match with the continuing desire to vape.

WITH EASYWAY, YOU REMOVE THE DESIRE COMPLETELY

The simplest of tasks becomes difficult if you go about it the wrong way. Opening a door, for example. You know how to open a door – you push on the handle and it swings open with the minimum of effort. But have you ever come across a door with no handle and pushed on the wrong side, where the hinges are? You're met with firm resistance. The door might budge a tiny bit, but it won't swing open. It requires a huge amount of effort and determination. Push on the correct side and the door opens without you even having to think about it.

Most vapers find it difficult to stop because they use the willpower method. They choose the difficult method because they've been brainwashed into believing that is the only way to quit. The method assumes that while the nicotine is leaving your body, you need to be strong-willed to get through two ordeals:

• the painful withdrawal period

• the sacrifice of your pleasure or crutch.

You should now be able to see the flaws in this theory. Firstly, there is no physical pain with nicotine withdrawal. Vapers go through it every moment that they're not vaping, every day of their vaping lives. You barely notice it.

The second flaw in the willpower theory is the assumption that quitting involves a sacrifice. This is only true if you regard vaping as your friend. But when you can see through the illusion that it gives you pleasure or a crutch and you know that nicotine does absolutely nothing for you whatsoever, there is no sense of sacrifice.

Whenever the thought of vaping enters your mind, you don't mope because you can't do it any more; you rejoice because you no longer have to. You're not 'giving up' anything when you quit – you're *getting rid* of something that's plagued your life.

TIGHTENING THE ROPE

People who try to quit with the willpower method constantly endure the tug-of-war of fear. You kill the Little Monster but leave the Big Monster alive. On one side, your rational brain knows you should stop because it's making you feel strange, costing you a fortune, controlling your life and making you miserable. On the other side your addicted brain makes you panic at the thought of being deprived of your pleasure or crutch. If you follow the willpower method, you focus on all the reasons for stopping and hope that if you can last long enough without doing it the desire will eventually go.

Some people do manage to quit through sheer force of will, but they don't become happy non-vapers. They never actually break free of their addiction, and so they are always fighting the temptation to fall back into the pit.

In most cases, the willpower method fails and you end up feeling more helpless and miserable than before.

With the willpower method, the struggle never ends. It becomes an ordeal, like running a marathon – except there is no finish line. You're forever waiting for something NOT to happen, so you never feel the elation of knowing you're free. With Easyway, you know you're a happy non-vaper the moment you kill the Big Monster and have your final dose of nicotine.

As long as you continue to believe that you're giving something up, you will always be running in pain. The stronger your will, the longer you will withstand the agony.

The longer you go on suffering a sense of deprivation, the more powerful your craving for nicotine becomes.

The feeling of deprivation makes you miserable, which in turn increases your desire for the drug – the crutch you always used to turn to in a crisis. You only have to succumb to this temptation once and all that hard work is wasted. Worse still, once you've failed on the willpower method, it's even harder to try again.

Failing to quit with the willpower method leaves you more addicted than before because it reinforces the belief that it is impossible to cure your problem. People will tell you they felt an enormous sense of relief when they gave in and had that first vape after an attempt to quit, but this relief is nothing more than a temporary end to the self-inflicted pain.

Nobody thinks, 'Great! I'm vaping again!' It is not a pleasure. In fact, it is accompanied by strong feelings of failure and foreboding, guilt and disappointment. Any hope you had that you might be free of the tyranny of nicotine is snuffed out in that moment.

If you believe that you lack the willpower to quit vaping, then you haven't yet understood the nature of the trap you're in. The more you will yourself to quit, the more you build up the belief that you're depriving yourself of something precious, and so the more you crave the very thing you're trying to give up.

This is how the rope tightens, keeping you firmly imprisoned. The only way to break the bonds is to understand the nature of the nicotine trap, let go of the struggle and unravel the brainwashing.

In other words:

> **YOU DON'T NEED WILL POWER, YOU JUST**
> **NEED TO KILL THE BIG MONSTER**

HOW WEAK-WILLED ARE YOU?

If you have tried and failed to quit in the past, did you put it down to a lack of willpower? Because the willpower method is so widely promoted, vapers don't question the validity behind it. You just assume that your failure to quit must be a flaw in you rather than the method. Believe me:

> **TELLING SOMEONE TO QUIT WITH THE WILLPOWER METHOD IS LIKE**
> **TELLING THEM TO OPEN A DOOR BY PUSHING ON THE HINGES**

Ask yourself whether you're weak-willed in other ways. Perhaps you drink or eat too much and you regard this as further evidence of a weak will. There is a connection between all addictions, but it's not that they are signs of a lack of willpower. On the contrary, they are more likely evidence of a strong will. What they all share is that they are traps created by misleading information and untruths. And one of the most misleading untruths is that quitting requires willpower.

In fact, most vapers, like smokers, are stubbornly strong-willed. It takes a strong-willed person to persist in doing something that goes against all their instincts. You know that vaping is dragging you further and further into the pit, making you increasingly stressed and unhappy, threatening to destroy your life, and yet you continue to do it.

The biggest fear for any drug addict is running out of their supply of the drug. Vapers go to incredible lengths to make sure they have a supply of nicotine at all times. This requires tremendous organisation, forethought and determination. Drug addicts are also determined liars. They will go way beyond the point of reason to deny their vaping to others and to themselves.

It also takes a strong will to persist in following a method that patently doesn't work. If I saw you trying to open a door by pushing on the hinges and I told you you'd find it easier if you pushed on the handle, but you ignored me and insisted on pushing on the hinges, I'd call you wilful, not weak-willed.

Think of all the people you know who are vapers. There are enough nicotine addicts in positions of power to illustrate that the addiction is not exclusive to the weak-willed. World leaders, captains of industry, entertainers, doctors... we have more people from the medical profession coming to Easyway for help than from any other walk of life. All of them reached their position in life through determination and hard work. In other words, they have immense willpower. So why would their willpower fail them when they try to stop doing something they think is destroying their health and controlling their life?

In fact, it tends to be the people with the strongest wills who find it hardest to quit by using the willpower method. Why? Because when the door fails to open, they won't give up and try to find an easier method; they'll force themselves to keep pushing on the hinges until they can push no more.

BEWARE OTHER QUITTERS

People who try to quit by the willpower method can have a harmful effect on your own desire to quit. They either brag about the sacrifices they're making or they whine about them. Either way, they reinforce the false belief that quitting demands a sacrifice.

THE BRAGGERS ARE EASY TO SPOT

They're the ones who become holier than thou anti-vaping zealots the moment they quit. Up go the 'No Smoking or Vaping' signs in their homes and cars. They'll invite you round just so they can forbid you to vape. And gloat.

They will take great delight in reminding you that by vaping you are damaging your health and it's costing you a fortune and they will tell you how they find it incomprehensible that an intelligent person like you still finds reasons to do it. Of course, they've conveniently forgotten that they spent years doing the very same thing.

Ex-vapers who have quit through willpower are far more vitriolic in their attacks on vaping than people who have never done it. Why are they so angry? Because beneath all that bragging and bluster they have not overcome their addiction. They still believe that they've made a sacrifice and they resent anyone who continues to feed their addiction.

Beware of the braggers; they can have a very negative effect on vapers who are thinking of quitting. Their bullying can drive you into the arms of your little crutch and make you lose sight of the real enemy. But worse than that, they reinforce the belief that: 'Once a nicotine addict, always a nicotine addict.' It's obvious that they still crave nicotine, so they create the impression that you can stop vaping but you can't escape.

THE WHINERS CONFIRM THIS IMPRESSION

Whiners will be the first to congratulate you when you have your last vape and throw out all your devices and juice. They will shake your hand, wish you success, fuel your elation by telling you how much healthier and wealthier you'll be, that you've made a really important decision and will never regret it... and then bring you crashing down by telling you how they quit years ago but still miss it terribly.

It can be enough to send you scrambling to rescue your vaping gear from the rubbish bin.

The last thing you want to hear when you're trying to quit is that you'll still be craving years from now. The good news is you won't. Braggers and whiners only continue to crave nicotine because they haven't killed the Big Monster. They have followed the wrong method and so they have nothing to offer you from their experience.

This is your sixth instruction, and it's important:

SIXTH INSTRUCTION: IGNORE ANY ADVICE
THAT GOES AGAINST EASYWAY

In particular, ignore the advice of anyone who claims to have quit by the willpower method. The fact is there is no sacrifice. Nicotine is NOT your friend so you are not 'giving up' anything.

People who quit with the willpower method are always waiting for the moment when the struggle ends and they become a happy non-vaper. But because the Big Monster is still alive, there is no finish line, no point in time when they stop wishing they could vape.

CROSSING THE LINE THE EASY WAY

With Easyway, there is nothing to wait for. You become a happy non-vaper the moment you unravel all the illusions that have led you into the nicotine trap, free yourself from fear and stop vaping with a feeling of excitement and elation. The elation of crossing the finish line occurs as soon as you remove the fear and illusions and stop vaping. That's when you kill the Big Monster and walk free from the addiction that has kept you enslaved. You need to understand that you will NOT get to that line by forcing yourself to suffer.

The psychology of the addict is such that a hard-line approach will not work. Rather than helping you to quit, it actually encourages you to stay hooked because:

IT REINFORCES THE MYTH THAT QUITTING IS HARD AND, THEREFORE, ADDS TO YOUR FEAR.

IT CREATES A FEELING OF DEPRIVATION, WHICH YOU WILL SEEK TO ALLEVIATE IN YOUR USUAL WAY – YOU WILL FALL BACK INTO THE TRAP.

You only need willpower if you have a conflict of will. We are going to resolve that conflict by removing one side of the tug-of-war of fear, so that all your will is going against vaping. Using willpower for the rest of your life to try not to vape is unlikely to prove successful and will not make you happy. Removing the need and desire to vape will.

Chapter 8

ADDICTIVE PERSONALITY THEORY

IN THIS CHAPTER
•A CONVENIENT EXCUSE •VAPERS WHO FAIL TO ESCAPE
•DEGREES OF ADDICTION •LIES, DAMNED LIES AND STATISTICS
•EFFECT NOT CAUSE

The addictive personality theory is just that – a theory. The belief that some people are more prone to addiction than others because of the way they're made stems from looking at the situation from the wrong perspective. The traits shared by addicts are not the cause of their addiction; they are the result.

A CONVENIENT EXCUSE

We're all agreed that there is a complete absence of logic in filling your lungs with poisonous vape. This is why vapers are constantly making feeble excuses to justify why they do it:

> 'It helps me relax.'
> 'I've got a lot of stress at the moment. I'll stop when things get easier.'
> 'It's my life. I'm allowed one little indulgence.'

We've established that all of these excuses are founded on the myth that vaping provides some sort of pleasure or crutch. But even when all the usual excuses have been shot down in flames and it's pointed out that their real reason for vaping is nicotine addiction, there is one last desperate plea that some vapers fall back on to justify their decision not to tackle their addiction.

'I HAVE AN ADDICTIVE PERSONALITY'

They've been led to believe that there's something in their genetic make-up that makes them more susceptible than most people to becoming hooked, and this makes it harder for them to escape. Of course, it suits them to believe this. It's a convenient excuse, but not one that will do them any good. Believe in the theory of the addictive personality and all you do is ensure that you remain forever trapped.

Sadly, their misconception is backed up by a number of so-called 'experts', who support the theory of the addictive personality. The term is bandied about so often that it's easy to be fooled into believing it's an established condition. It is not. It's a theory, largely based on the fact that a number of addicts are addicted to more than one thing: for example, drinkers who are also smokers or vapers or gamblers, or heroin addicts who smoke or vape and are heavily in debt.

But all addictions involve the same kind of trap, so it's obvious that someone who is susceptible to one addiction will be susceptible to others. It's nothing to do with genetics; it's all to do with not understanding the trap and believing the myth that these things give you a genuine pleasure or crutch. Remember:

THE MISERY OF ADDICTION IS NOT RELIEVED BY THE
THING YOU ARE ADDICTED TO – IT'S CAUSED BY IT

VAPERS WHO FAIL TO ESCAPE

The fear of success drives addicts to seek reasons to avoid even trying to quit. The addictive personality theory gives them the perfect excuse. If you think you have an addictive personality, you will regard quitting as an impossible task. 'How can I override my own genetic make-up?' This illusion can also be reinforced by your failed attempts to quit by using willpower.

It is further confirmed by people who have quit by using the willpower method and are feeling deprived because they still believe they're making a sacrifice – the braggers and whiners we covered earlier. If they've abstained for years and are still craving their little crutch, and we've established that it's nothing to do with willpower, it's tempting to believe that there must be some flaw in their genetic make-up that keeps drawing them back.

But there is another explanation:

THEY'VE BEEN CONNED

Braggers and whiners are still labouring under the illusion that they are making a genuine sacrifice. Their willpower is pulling them in opposite directions: they desperately want to satisfy their craving, yet they desperately want to be a non-vaper too. They are caught up in the tug-of-war of fear and eventually they lose – all because of an illusion.

We've established that you are not 'giving up' anything. This gives you an enormous advantage over the braggers and whiners. Make sure you're not fooled by the illusion that keeps them in the trap.

Pleading an addictive personality is just another excuse for doing something that you know is completely illogical. You don't want to stay enslaved by the Big Monster, with all the fear, misery and sickness that goes with it. That's why you're reading this book. You have made the decision to escape and you are well on the way to doing just that.

Escape is easy, provided you keep an open mind. If you cling to the excuse that you have an addictive personality, it means that your mind is not open and you risk sentencing yourself to remaining enslaved for the rest of your life.

When you keep trying and failing to quit, you end up feeling stupid and helpless. Putting your addiction down to a flaw in your personality can appear to be the rational explanation you need. With Easyway, you discover the real explanation. The spread of misinformation is so relentless that anybody can be conned and most people *are* to some extent, even non-vapers. You weren't stupid to get hooked and neither were the millions of other vapers. Neither are you stupid or weak for being unable to quit. You've just been following the wrong method.

Once you see the true picture of how addiction works, the illusions disappear and you realise that you are complete without your little crutch.

WITH IT, YOU ARE A SLAVE

DEGREES OF ADDICTION

So why do some people fall deeper into the trap than others? Why can one person have the occasional vape, while another ends up puffing away all day and night, every day and night? Doesn't that suggest that one is more prone to addiction than the other?

Well, yes, it does, but why should that have anything to do with their personality? There are numerous differences between people, which can explain why one is prone to vaping more than another. Everyone reading this now will vape different amounts due to different circumstances, such as money and opportunity, but all of you feel the same way about vaping and are trying to find the same solution: to escape.

Some aren't physically equipped to vape more and so have to limit their intake accordingly. Others have jobs that mean they can't vape as much as they might do if they had more leisure, and others simply can't afford it.

Our behaviour is largely affected by the influences we are subjected to as we grow up: different parents, teachers, friends, things we read, watch and listen to, places we go, people we meet, etc. All of these factors will have a bearing on how quickly we descend into the trap and they vary for everybody. But they are all controllable and reversible. They have nothing to do with genetics or anything fixed in our personality. Be quite clear:

ANYBODY CAN FALL INTO THE NICOTINE TRAP
AND ANYBODY CAN ESCAPE JUST AS EASILY

LIES, DAMNED LIES AND STATISTICS

Addiction is a lonely place. Despite the knowledge that millions of people in the world are suffering from the same addiction, vapers and all other addicts think that their own problem is unique to them. When you come out of your cocoon and speak to people about your problems, you discover that they are experiencing, or have experienced, exactly what you are going through. Then you begin to see that addiction is not a weakness in the individual, but a weakness in the society that brainwashes individuals into the trap.

Next time you have to go outside to vape, pay attention to the other vapers or smokers out there with you. Birds of a feather flock together and vapers and smokers certainly appear to be flocking when you see them huddled together in the rain outside their workplaces, 'enjoying' nicotine. As a vaper or smoker there is a sense that you're a different breed from everyone else. You appear to share similar character traits with other vapers or smokers and you feel more comfortable in their company.

The temptation is to believe that these traits are evidence of a shared personality – an addictive personality that led you to become addicted to nicotine. The reality is that they are the *result* of nicotine addiction.

The reason addicts feel more comfortable in the company of similar addicts is not because they're more interesting or fun; on the contrary, the attraction lies in the very fact that they won't challenge you or make you think twice about your addiction because they're in the same boat. All addicts know that they're doing something stupid and self-destructive. If you're surrounded by other people doing the same thing, you don't feel quite so foolish. Although no doubt there are smokers out there who try to make vapers feel foolish and vapers who try to make smokers look foolish.

The good news is that once you're free from the addiction you also get free from the harmful effects it has on your character.

The belief that you were doomed from birth to be a nicotine addict will be self-fulfilling if you allow it to remain in your mind. Think about it logically. The addictive personality theory is based on statistics, but if you examine the statistics closely they actually make the likelihood of an addictive gene appear far-fetched.

If there was an addictive gene, you would expect the percentage of addicts in the world to have remained fairly constant throughout history. Yet in less than a century, the incidence of nicotine addiction has changed dramatically. In 1948 82 per cent of the UK adult male population were smokers; today it's less than 20 per cent. A similar trend is evident throughout the USA and most of Western Europe and Australasia. So are we to conclude that the proportion of people with addictive personalities has fallen by around 75 per cent in just over half a century? That's a major genetic shift in mankind!

At the same time, the number of smokers in Asia has soared. What complex genetic anomaly is this that rises and falls so rapidly, and even appears to transfer itself wholesale from one continent to another? And, more to the point, with reference to the so-called JUUL epidemic in the USA, was there suddenly a genetic bump in the number of people predisposed to becoming addicted to nicotine? Or isn't the following true? That a generation of kids has been allowed to fall easy prey to one of the smartest, most sophisticated, psychopathic marketing machines on the planet:

THE NICOTINE INDUSTRY

It doesn't really matter if you believe you have an addictive personality or gene anyway – the fact is that it is easy to get free just as long as you know how, regardless of whether you have an addictive personality or gene or not.

EFFECT NOT CAUSE

It's essential that you understand that you didn't become addicted to nicotine because you have an addictive personality. If you think you have an addictive personality, it's simply because of the fact that you got addicted to nicotine.

This is the trick that addiction plays on you. It makes you feel that you're dependent on your addiction and that there's some weakness in your character or genetic make-up. It distorts your perceptions and thereby maintains its grip on you.

The addictive personality theory encourages the belief that escape is out of your hands and that you are condemned to a life of slavery and misery. Remember, you didn't feel the need or desire to vape until you started doing it. It was vaping that created the addiction, not the other way around.

When you finish this book the misery and slavery of nicotine addiction will be behind you. Once you have stripped away all the illusions and can see the situation in its true light without any doubts whatsoever, you'll wonder how you were ever conned into seeing it differently. But like millions of people around the world, you have been the victim of an ingenious trap. Recognise the trap for what it is, dismiss the idea of a flaw in your personality and you will be ready to walk free.

Just keep an open mind and keep following all the instructions.

Chapter 9

CONQUERING CONCENTRATION

IN THIS CHAPTER

• *A BRAINWASHED BELIEF* • *NO OPTION, NO DISTRACTION*
• *IT'S NOT A WEIGHTY MATTER* • *THE TRUTH INITIATIVE*
• *TV IS SO YESTERDAY!* • *REBEL WITHOUT A CAUSE*
• *SO WHAT ABOUT THE WEIGHT ISSUE?* • *DEPRESSION AND SELF-HARM*
• *HOW TO CONCENTRATE* • *BORING BORING VAPING*
• *FREEDOM FROM BRAINWASHING* • *ACHIEVING CERTAINTY*

Nicotine propaganda has built the drug up over the years so it appears to be the solution to almost any problem. The image of Sherlock Holmes puffing away on his pipe as he tries to crack his latest case has become a symbol for another of the great myths: that nicotine helps you concentrate. It's essential that you remove this belief from your mind before you quit. It's embarrassing in our live seminars when a vaper or smoker cites Sherlock as an example of an intellectual high achiever who used nicotine. It never occurs to them, until we gently point it out, that of course Holmes is an entirely fictional character. He never existed.

A BRAINWASHED BELIEF

Up until now you have been encouraged not to change your normal vaping pattern because we don't want you to suffer any distractions while you're progressing through the book. You may have interpreted this to mean that continuing to vape will help you concentrate. Believe me, it means nothing of the sort.

VAPING DESTROYS CONCENTRATION

Nicotine addicts are brainwashed into believing that it aids concentration, and the back-to-front nature of the trap appears to confirm the fact. Until you remove this belief from your mind, you will find it hard to concentrate if you're craving a vape. So have a vape when you feel the craving and continue to read the book without worrying about it.

We all have times, whether in our work or our home life, when we need to focus on a problem and we don't relish the thought. For vapers, this is a common trigger for reaching for a vape. You believe that vaping can do two things: relieve the anxiety of confronting the problem and help you to rally your thoughts into finding a solution. As soon as this belief is planted in your mind, it becomes impossible to concentrate. No matter how hard you try to concentrate on the problem, the thought that a vape will make the situation better becomes an increasing distraction.

Eventually you cave in and vape. The anxiety disappears and you find the answer you've been looking for. Naturally you conclude that the vape has made all the difference. You needed to vape to be able to concentrate. So far, so predictable.

• **You believed vaping would help you concentrate.**

• **You vaped.**

• **You found the concentration you needed...**

• **What's the problem?**

The problem is that it's an illusion – one that's keeping you in the nicotine trap, controlling your life and stealing your money. So what really happened?

• **You believed vaping would help you concentrate.**

• **You became obsessed with the idea, so you were unable to concentrate until you vaped.**

• **The vape appeared to solve the problem but it actually caused it.**

It's like someone stealing the tiles off your roof and then coming around and offering to sell them back to you the very next day.

Non-vapers don't suffer the distraction of craving nicotine, a craving that is only partially relieved by having a vape. And neither do they poison their body and brain as you do every time you vape, so their ability to think clearly and creatively is not hampered.

Not only does vaping cause a distraction when you least want one (when you're not able to vape), but when you're able to vape you're not even aware that you're doing it, let alone distracted by it. It also destroys your ability to concentrate.

NO OPTION, NO DISTRACTION

When we're faced with a problem we don't like, we seek comfort in distractions because they delay the dreaded moment when we have to get to grips with the problem. Some people make a cup of tea, some make themselves something to eat, some check their emails or look at their phone. We convince ourselves that there's value in doing these things because that gives us the excuse to put off the inevitable.

But none of these things help to solve the problem. In fact, they only make it worse. Leave a problem unsolved and it will usually get bigger. It certainly won't go away. But as long as we have the belief that any of these things will help, we won't be able to tackle the problem properly until we do them. Vaping is just another self-imposed distraction. It's not the physical craving for nicotine that prevents us from being able to concentrate, because that craving is almost indiscernible. It's the mental obsession caused by the Big Monster.

You can prove your own ability to concentrate without nicotine by putting yourself in a situation where vaping is not an option. A good example is an exam room. Every year countless students sit their finals. A proportion of them are vapers, who are used to studying with a vape on the go. When it dawns on them that they are going to have to sit through hours in an exam room without vaping, panic sets in. They try sitting a practice paper without vaping and find their hands shaking so much they can't write!

Yet when it comes to the exam proper, most of them sit through it without the thought of vaping ever entering their heads. It's clear that they are perfectly capable of concentrating for several hours without their little crutch.

So what makes all the difference? Quite simply the fact that vaping was never an option in the exam room, so it never became a distraction.

When you know you can't have something it's easy to put it out of your mind. Millions of smokers, followed by vapers, have discovered this since smoking and vaping was banned on planes and trains. What would once have been a dreaded situation is no problem at all because they don't spend the journey moping for something they can't have. They can put the thought right out of their minds until they have reached their destination.

Actually, let me digress for a few moments here, because I'd like to recap on how weak nicotine addiction is and there's a great example involving a vaper on a flight that illustrates it perfectly.

Consider a heavy vaper on a long-haul flight who cannot vape.

The vaper becomes resigned to this fact. Most vapers – even the heaviest in these circumstances – don't even bother using nicotine patches or gum.

For most of the flight, the vaper feels calm. Yet, 10 hours into an 11-hour flight, something begins to happen. The flight is coming to an end and the vaper begins to anticipate getting off the plane and being able to vape as much as they want.

When the vaper checks the time and notes there is now only the small matter of 20 minutes until the end of the flight, a smile appears on the vaper's face.

Now imagine that vaper when the flight's captain announces that due to severe weather conditions at their destination the flight has been diverted to a different airport and the journey will now last a further 60 minutes.

Wow! All of a sudden the calm disappears, along with the smile, from the vaper's face. The vaper lurches into a condition that they would immediately describe as nicotine withdrawal: anger, tension, anxiety, upset and stress. Nicotine withdrawal didn't just happen in the six seconds that it took the pilot to announce the delayed landing. It has been occurring continuously since the vaper last vaped more than 10 hours and 40 minutes ago.

But nicotine withdrawal did not cause the sudden onset of unpleasant symptoms.

Something in the vaper's mind changed as a result of the pilot's announcement: it was the Big Monster.

If you're dismissing this story because you feel any self-respecting vaper would get around the problem by vaping discreetly in the bathrooms, or even under a blanket, then you're in danger of missing the point. Don't worry – if you understand the point simply on principle, that's all you need to do.

IT'S NOT A WEIGHTY MATTER

One of the most common misconceptions about vaping is that it plays a part in helping to control weight.

There are several factors involved in this illusion: the belief that vaping acts as an appetite suppressant, enabling vapers to skip meals and snacks (substituting food for vaping); the idea that vaping burns calories by increasing the addict's metabolic rate; and the relentless influence of the nicotine industry, which continues the work it started years ago by portraying glamorous, svelte stars smoking and vaping.

Big Nicotine has infiltrated the fashion and music industries and continues to manipulate the film industry.

Young bands, solo performers and sports stars continue to have their images used in adverts and sponsorship tours across the globe. And in countries where advertising is banned, they influence the inclusion of vaping and smoking in photo shoots, and paparazzi shots in newspapers. The fashion industry is the most blatant in its cosy arrangements with the tobacco and vaping giants, with cigarettes and vaping frequently appearing on the fashion show runways and in glossy shoots for magazines.

Hollywood is always eager to assist too. There are many examples of leading characters being portrayed as smokers and vapers, sometimes, bizarrely, even in films set hundreds of years into the future. It's always the same message: nicotine is cool, nicotine is tough and, even more important, nicotine will survive.

No wonder by the time a potential vaper reaches an age whereby they might be tempted to try it, they're already convinced that it's a cool, sophisticated, stylish, sexy thing to do, with the added benefit that it's also some kind of magical means of controlling weight.

You're not an idiot; you don't need me to tell you that those sexy, glamorous, stylish and sophisticated stars weren't made to look that way by cigarettes or JUUL or IQOS or any other nicotine device. It was the other way around: the stars made the nicotine devices appear sexy, glamorous, stylish and sophisticated. Nicotine just isn't sexy!

THE TRUTH INITIATIVE

Studies and reports by The Truth Initiative state that 86 per cent of the 2018 Oscar nominees in major categories featured tobacco or vaping imagery on screen.

PG-rated films on the Oscar list feature twice as much smoking as in 2017 and they've already delivered 2.5 times more tobacco impressions to cinema audiences. Of the 2019 Oscar-nominated films that were rated PG-13, the ones that had the most smoking included *Bohemian Rhapsody* (152 tobacco incidents) and *Green Book* (381 tobacco incidents). Tobacco use in streaming series such as *Stranger Things*, *House of Cards* and *Orange is the*

New Black is pervasive and more prominent than it is in broadcast content.

Seventy-nine per cent of the shows most popular with young people, aged 15–24 years, depict smoking prominently, the research finds. The critically acclaimed *Stranger Things*, nominated for two Golden Globe Awards in 2018, including best television drama series, has emerged as the worst offender. The Netflix hit, which won five Creative Arts Emmy Awards in 2017 and drew an estimated 15.8 million viewers within three days of its second-season launch, features more than 180 tobacco incidents in the 2016 season. It is followed by *Orange is the New Black* (45 incidents) and *House of Cards* (41 incidents). Other Netflix shows analysed in the research include *Making a Murderer*, *Fuller House*, *Unbreakable Kimmy Schmidt* and *Daredevil*. Sometimes you may feel that the number of nicotine-related incidents is low, such as in *House of Cards*, but this doesn't present the full picture. The way in which cigarettes, smoking and vaping have been portrayed as being hugely desirable, highly sexualised and an essential, albeit rare, 'treat' does powerful work for Big Nicotine in the minds of young people.

TV IS *SO* YESTERDAY!

It's not just traditional TV, streaming services such as Netflix, or mainstream films that are leading the onslaught against our youngsters – social media is awash with every kind of e-cigarette, vaping, JUULing and smoking propaganda imaginable and some which you'd struggle to even imagine. Young, beautiful people earn big money by promoting any number of brands of nicotine addiction – without restriction and without the viewers/followers even knowing that the influential social media starlet has been paid to big up the products.

Tobacco use is also widespread in video games, including those rated appropriate for teenagers, but tobacco warnings are not. Many of the top games include the glamourisation of smoking or vaping.

Let's look at JUUL. In December 2018, US Surgeon General Jerome M. Adams declared e-cigarette use among teenagers an 'epidemic' in the USA and Health and Human Services Secretary Alex Azar stated: 'In the data sets we use, we have never seen use of any substance by America's young people rise as rapidly as e-cigarette use is rising.'

These are simply unprecedented increases.

In 2019 JUUL was estimated to be worth a staggering $38 billion. That alone is extraordinary, but when you appreciate that the company didn't exist until 2017 it's simply mind-boggling.

They're very good at sales and marketing, have deliberately targeted youngsters and their growth, of course, is greatly assisted by the fact that their product is highly addictive. A lifetime of addiction awaits those who do not know how to get free and the gateway effect (vaping leading to smoking) is firmly becoming established.

Aside from that, it will be many years before the true harm that vaping causes is known. It's a nicotine time bomb.

REBEL WITHOUT A CAUSE

Then there's the myth of the vaping rebel. There are a million ways of rebelling, none of which involve being a pathetic victim of an awful addiction. You choose to rebel; you don't choose whether you vape or not. There is truly nothing sadder than a vaper who claims they're doing it for this reason – deep down inside, not even they believe it. They know that, far from vaping being rebellious, they're simply doing it because they're enslaved.

SO WHAT ABOUT THE WEIGHT ISSUE?

Firstly, you know yourself, you see plenty of overweight vapers. If vaping was that efficient, surely that wouldn't be the case? More importantly, if that was the case, the more someone vaped the skinnier they'd be – but heavy vapers tend to be the most overweight of all.

Vaping does indeed increase your metabolic rate, the rate at which your body burns calories. Glossy fitness magazines hark on endlessly about this. What they don't tell their readers is that the impact of vaping on your metabolic rate is insignificant in terms of weight control. Think how hard and long you have to pedal on an exercise bike at the gym to burn off a few hundred calories. There simply isn't this fat-burning, calorie-burning process going on in your body as a result of your vaping.

Another favourite myth of glossy magazines is that vaping acts as an appetite suppressant. It seems to make sense to us as vapers. We get hungry, have a vape and the hunger goes. In our mind it's the vape that's magically taken away our hunger. What we don't realise is that when a non-vaper ignores hunger for a couple of minutes, their hunger also disappears. Non-vapers don't give the credit for this to vaping; but for vapers, it confirms the myth that vaping suppresses appetite. They ignore the fact that when they experience more severe hunger a vape won't do the trick. And it never did.

Pick up your vape liquid. Examine the labelling carefully. Can you find the text that says, 'Used as part of a calorie-controlled diet this e-liquid will help you control weight'? Of course, nothing of the sort is written on the label. Why not?

BECAUSE IT'S NOT TRUE

If it was, the nicotine industry would be allowed to write it on the packaging and no one could stop them.

So how have we become so convinced that vaping helps with weight control? It's failed attempts by ourselves and others to quit vaping using willpower that causes the problem. If it hasn't happened to you, it will have happened to someone you know. Smokers or vapers quit and put on weight. Why? They haven't killed the Big Monster and therefore constantly feel deprived.

In an attempt to get rid of the desire to vape and the feeling of deprivation that they suffer, they tend to eat or drink in place of vaping. It doesn't really work, but nevertheless they carry on and naturally gain weight as a result. When they finally cave in and vape again, they stop overeating and the weight seems to drop off. It confirms the myth, meaning the fear of gaining weight stays with them and puts them off ever trying to quit again.

This doesn't happen with Easyway. Why not? Because Easyway removes the desire to vape. If there is no desire to vape, there is no feeling of deprivation, and there is no need or compulsion to substitute (eat or drink instead of vape).

You won't be inclined to substitute when you quit vaping with Easyway, so there is no need for you to gain weight. Far from it, you'll be so full of energy you'll be glowing with good health.

I'll talk more about the link between vaping and hunger later, but for the time being I will just say that if you're concerned about weight gain, rest assured it simply isn't going to happen this time.

You won't cure a weight problem by vaping; neither will you cause one when you quit using Easyway.

DEPRESSION AND SELF-HARM

We receive letters and emails every week from nicotine addicts all over the world asking for clarification on certain points.

Be reassured that as a result of all this correspondence, you're reading the most up-to-date and comprehensive version of Allen Carr's Easyway method to date.

Two issues that arise with a small number of correspondents are those relating to acute/chronic depression and self-harm. These are two quite separate issues; nevertheless, I'm happy to handle them in the same section. Nicotine addicts who live with those conditions are concerned that Easyway may not work for them. Those suffering with severe depression sense that vaping or smoking helps them deal with the problem in some way. In fact, it's quite the reverse. Nicotine addiction has been proven to cause and exacerbate depression rather than ease it, so please rest assured. If you live with that extremely challenging condition, Easyway will still work for you. Any belief that vaping or smoking or using nicotine in any form helps you deal with your depression is understandable but it is no different from anyone who believes, for example, that vaping helps them cope with stress. You can relate to every part of the method – and just as we're fooled into believing that vaping helps us cope with stress, so we are fooled into believing it helps us cope with depression.

As far as self-harm is concerned, a vaper or smoker might say something to the effect of: 'I do it to punish myself or hurt myself or because I don't care about myself.' If you harbour those beliefs, you need to understand that you don't vape because it harms you; you do it because you are addicted to nicotine.

On some level, you may be choosing to self-harm in other ways, yet you have no choice as to whether you vape or not. In this way, you're no different from any nicotine addict on this planet.

Self-harm may well have been the motivation to start vaping or smoking, but remember we all started for a variety of phoney and foolish reasons; whether it was to be part of the gang, or the opposite, to go against the flow and rebel, to try to look tough, cool or sophisticated, just out of sheer curiosity, or to show the world that we didn't care. The fact is that the reason we start vaping has no bearing on why we then continue to do it, nor does it prevent us from stopping.

There are many more effective, efficient and significant ways of self-harming, if that is what you wish to do. Vaping is entirely un-satisfactory in that regard since it takes years, sometimes decades, to get what might be described as the self-harm pay-off. People who want to self-harm do it immediately and painfully. Put simply, self-harm isn't why you vape.

It might be one of the reasons you tried vaping in the first place, and it might be an excuse you use to justify the fact that you have carried on doing it or to excuse yourself for your failure to quit, but it simply is not why you vape. To claim otherwise implies that you have some kind of choice or control over vaping. If you had any choice over whether you vape or not, you wouldn't be reading this book. Don't get me wrong. Perhaps in the past, when you fell back into vaping after a period of freedom, you did so with an attitude of 'So what – I don't care if I live or die!', but at that point you didn't throw yourself off a cliff. In that situation, it's no more than a phoney justification for returning to nicotine addiction. The real reason for the return to vaping was the belief that it does something for you.

The great news is that because self-harm isn't why you've been vaping, you have no need to swap vaping as a means of hurting yourself for any other self-harming activity once you've quit. People who live with depression and genuine self-harming issues do so with amazing strength and resilience and deserve our respect and admiration. The wonderful news is that, no matter what highs or lows might befall you once you've quit, I can assure you that the highs will be higher and the lows will be less intense and easier to handle.

HOW TO CONCENTRATE

The first thing you need to do in order to concentrate on anything is remove all distractions. If someone's making a distracting noise, you can ask them to stop or you can move to somewhere quiet. But say you're the one causing the distraction – perhaps you have a cold and are constantly sniffing. It's a distraction, but what can you do about it? Nothing, so you just put it out of your mind and focus on the job in hand.

If there is something you can do to remove a distraction, you need to do it, or else it will irritate you and that will become an added distraction. If there is nothing you can do about it, it's much easier to ignore it and put it out of your mind. When you have a choice, you have to make a decision. Until you make that decision, you will be distracted by the choice. Take away the choice and you take away the pressure to make a decision.

Perhaps you think I'm suggesting that enforced denial is the key to quitting vaping permanently. Absolutely not. But the way vapers are able to get by quite happily when vaping is not an option does prove that it's easy to put vaping out of your mind, even when you're still hooked.

The problem for vapers is that the option to do it is available most of the time. When you try to quit with the willpower method, you are always aware of that option and always distracted by it. With Easyway, you remove the option to vape. Not by denying yourself JUUL, or IQOS or any other nicotine device, but by removing all desire to take the drug.

For non-vapers, vaping is never a serious option – and it won't be for you when you reach the end of this book.

BORING BORING VAPING

Closely associated with the concentration myth is the myth that vaping helps to alleviate boredom. Again, this myth is created by the back-to-front nature of the trap. When your brain is not stimulated you have nothing to take your mind off the cries of the Little Monster, and so you tend to scratch the itch.

Vaping becomes your default response to boredom. But it doesn't remove the boredom.

Boredom is relieved by occupying your mind with something interesting. The exam room scenario proves that vapers can go for long periods without doing it and don't even think about it when their minds are occupied. But there's nothing interesting about vaping. When you're taking a drag of that toxic vapour, are you really thinking: 'This is fascinating!' There are few more tediously repetitive activities than vaping, again and again, day in, day out. It may be a fascination at the very beginning, but it quickly becomes so boring that you're not even aware that you're doing it most of the time.

Take a close look at vapers or smokers next time you're stuck in traffic. They'll be vaping or smoking, but they'll be every bit as bored as everyone else in the jam. Look at the vapers huddled outside work taking one of their vape or smoking breaks. Do they look stimulated and happy? Or do they look bored and miserable?

Just as vaping destroys concentration, it also increases boredom by reducing your opportunities for physical and mental stimulation; thereby depleting your energy, making you sluggish, lethargic and lazy and destroying your zest for life. It's miserable being addicted to anything.

FREEDOM FROM BRAINWASHING

Nicotine addiction is a tyrant. Just when you think you're putting up a resistance to the desire to vape, something comes along that triggers the belief that you 'need' a vape and all your resistance crumbles. A typical trigger is a problem that demands your attention. Up go your stress levels and, because you've been brainwashed into believing that vaping relieves stress, you reach for nicotine.

So how can you avoid these triggers after you quit? Simple:

YOU DON'T NEED TO AVOID TRIGGERS

When you understand how the triggers work, they cease to be triggers. Everybody comes up against tricky problems from time to time. It's a fact of life. But not everybody reaches for a vape every time they're faced with a problem that demands concentration. Non-vapers don't see e-cigarettes as a crutch that will help them cope with the challenge and consequently they spend much less time agonising over problems.

The problem vapers have is that, in addition to the real-life problem that's facing them, they have the uncertainty about whether or not they should vape. So they have not one difficult decision to make but two. This delays the process of tackling the real problem, dragging it out and making it worse while they try to cope with the distraction of wondering whether to vape or not.

REMOVE THE DOUBT FROM A VAPER'S MIND AND QUITTING BECOMES EASY

There may come a time after you've had your final vape when you find yourself faced with a stressful problem and the thought enters your head to have a vape. It's important that you prepare yourself for this and are not alarmed. The thought is just a hangover from your vaping days. You don't have to go along with it. All you have to do is remind yourself of what you know to be the truth: vaping benefits you in no way whatsoever. You know you've made the right decision and no purpose will be served by delving into the subject.

Instead of feeling deprived, rejoice in the fact that you are now a non-vaper and you have no need to fall into the tyrant's trap.

People who quit with the willpower method spend the rest of their lives trying to avoid the triggers that used to make them reach for nicotine. They don't trust themselves to resist the temptation to vape if any of those triggers occur. When you have the certainty that vaping or JUULing or IQOSing or dipping or snusing does absolutely nothing for you whatsoever, there is no need to avoid the triggers because they no longer work as triggers.

Indeed, the triggers can serve to reinforce your sense of satisfaction and joy at having quit. Every time something happens that reminds you of when you used to vape, it acts as a truly enjoyable reminder that you are free.

ACHIEVING CERTAINTY

Removing the doubt and achieving the certainty you need is a simple process of looking at the facts and seeing things as they really are. Most vapers don't do this when they try to quit. They just look at the reasons for not doing it – the health risks, the wasted money, the smell, etc. – and hope that will be enough to overcome their desire to vape.

Of course, the Big Monster isn't going to be silenced by such concerns. If it was, no vaper would have any trouble quitting. In order to kill the Big Monster, you need to see vaping for what it really is –

a drug addiction that does nothing for you whatsoever – and allow understanding to replace brainwashing.

SEVENTH INSTRUCTION: HAVE NO DOUBT ABOUT YOUR DECISION TO QUIT

When you are certain that vaping does nothing for you, you will find that your desire to do it evaporates. The only reason anyone chooses to start vaping is because of the myth that it provides some sort of pleasure or crutch. Unravel the myth and you remove the desire.

You are now halfway to achieving your dream of being free from nicotine and becoming a happy non-vaper. I should add the word 'again', because you were free from the tyranny of addiction before you started vaping. You may have forgotten what it felt like. After your final vape, you will quickly rediscover the pleasures and benefits of being a non-vaper.

BETTER HEALTH

MORE MONEY

GREATER SELF-ESTEEM

In addition, you will discover the truth that has been hidden from you while you've been under the tyranny of nicotine addiction, that without nicotine you will be:

MORE RELAXED

MORE RESILIENT TO STRESS

BETTER ABLE TO CONCENTRATE

You will also enjoy all your meals more because your taste buds will regain their sensitivity and you'll be happy to take your time rather than rush to the end so you can vape. You will have the energy to get more out of exercise and sex. And best of all, you'll be free from the sense of slavery that leaves all vapers feeling helpless and stupid.

Soon you'll finish off the Big Monster. So enjoy the thought that you are taking steps to free yourself from the tyranny of nicotine addiction. And carry on vaping, or using whatever nicotine product you use. Don't feel guilty, don't be concerned about it – freedom awaits. All you need to do is follow the instructions.

WE ARE GOING TO DELIVER THE FINAL FATAL BLOWS TO THE BIG MONSTER. FREE YOUR MIND FROM ANY LINGERING BELIEF THAT VAPING PROVIDES YOU WITH ANY KIND OF PLEASURE OR CRUTCH AND SNUFF OUT YOUR DESIRE FOR NICOTINE ONCE AND FOR ALL.

On the way, we will examine more of the myths that keep nicotine addicts in the trap, including the theory that substitutes can help you get through the process of quitting by keeping you topped up with nicotine while you work on getting out of 'the habit'. Remember, you don't vape out of habit, you vape because you're hooked on nicotine. Keep taking nicotine – in any form – and you're going to stay hooked.

A lot of people are drawn to vaping, and a lot are therefore put off trying to quit, by the myth that vaping is a good way to keep your weight down.

We will look closely again at the connection between vaping or smoking and weight and explain why you will find it much easier to get in shape when you're not a slave to nicotine.

We will then look at the different types of vaper – the casual vapers, heavy vapers, stoppers and starters, etc. – and examine what, if anything, makes them different. You might be surprised by the conclusion. But if you're clear on everything you've read so far, you should already have guessed it.

By the end of this book you will be ready and eager to have your final vape, get rid of your device and vaping paraphernalia and get on with life as a happy non-vaper, but you might still have one or two burning questions that are making you feel uncertain. We need to eradicate all uncertainty when it comes to your decision to quit. So we will address all the lingering doubts, so that you are fully prepared to take that momentous step and walk free from the nicotine trap and have your final vape.

Congratulations on your achievements so far. You have come a very long way towards freeing yourself from the tyranny of vaping. Your mindset is already very different to how it was before you started this book. The myths that have kept you in the nicotine trap have started to unravel and you are moving closer and closer to destroying the Big Monster once and for all.

Perhaps you feel you have already destroyed it; in which case you're ahead of the game. That's great news, but beware!

Remember what I said about the instructions: you need to follow them all in order until the end. If you skip past any part of the book, you will not be following the method and you will miss out on a key step in your journey to freedom. This might not seem important now while you're full of zeal for quitting, but later you may be vulnerable to being dragged back into the trap if you don't follow the method in full.

So let's get on with it and take a close look at the way the Big Monster takes shape in your mind.

Chapter 10

SPREADING THE MYTH

IN THIS CHAPTER

*THE BIG CON *GETTING HOOKED *ALL VAPERS LIE
*LURING YOU BACK IN *THE MIRACLE OF UNCLE JACK
*THE RIGHT TO VAPE *FEAR *ROLE MODELS
*SEEING THE TRUTH TOO LATE

*It is perfectly possible for a man to be out of prison and
yet not free – to be under no physical constraint and yet
to be a psychological captive, compelled to think, feel and
act as the representatives of the national State, or of some
private interest within the nation, want him to think, feel
and act.*

Aldous Huxley, Brave New World

THE BIG CON

To use the words of Aldous Huxley, vapers, and in fact all nicotine
addicts, are 'psychological captives'. Perhaps you think I'm going
too far in comparing the world of nicotine addiction to the dystopian
world of Huxley's imagination. OK, nicotine is a highly addictive
drug, but surely I'm not suggesting that the tobacco industry and the
pharmaceutical industry, with the nicotine industry carved up between

them, are so evil as to trap their victims into a spiral of self-destruction by brainwashing them into believing their products are good for them, or at least not so bad for them!

Well, the tobacco industry can hardly be held up as a paragon of virtue. They are more and more involved in the vaping industry and have a history of lies, deceit and suppression of evidence that has cost tens of millions of lives. Furthermore, they continue to push out products that are proven to be the cause of more than seven million deaths every year worldwide. These people, and those under their influence – whether in politics or in the medical establishment – are responsible for the second great wave of nicotine addiction: vaping.

Ask yourself a few questions:

* **Can you trust them?**

* **Do you want to be controlled by them?**

* **Do you want your kids to be controlled by them?**

* **Are you comfortable putting the length, quality and enjoyment of your future life in their hands?**

Only you can answer those questions – although I suspect you already have. They're part of the reason that you're reading this book.

But there is something far more sinister at work. Even the nicotine industry is not clever enough to devise the level of brainwashing that leads millions of people to smoke or vape in spite of the obvious dangers and disadvantages. It doesn't have to.

SMOKERS AND VAPERS ARE ALREADY DOING
THE INDUSTRY'S DIRTY WORK

Nobody spreads the myths that con us into nicotine addiction more than the addicts themselves. It seems incredible, doesn't it? No smoker enjoys smoking, no vaper genuinely enjoys vaping, most of them wish they could stop, yet every nicotine addict promotes the belief that it provides some kind of pleasure or crutch.

The solution is simple – it's getting smokers and vapers to stop listening to each other and start hearing the truth about nicotine addiction that poses the challenge.

It's time for you to see the nicotine industry as it really is: an addiction business which is designed to enslave you for life. For life!!

You may be thinking that it's OK to call out the tobacco industry (they've been proven not to care), but surely I shouldn't be so tough on the pharmaceutical industry or new corporations involving themselves in the addiction business, such as JUUL. Don't they exist in order to do good? Aren't their products the result of their desire to cure smokers of their addiction? JUUL's merciless advertising and marketing strategy, targeting non-smoking youngsters throughout the USA over the first few years of their existence, puts paid to that myth.

The pharmaceutical industry per se does an awful lot of good. But it also does tremendous harm. Its manipulation of clinical trials is well chronicled. And if you observe the nature of the beast, you'll notice it's incentivised to find treatments rather than cures – preferably treatments that last a lifetime.

WHY WOULD THEY PREFER TO FIND
TREATMENTS RATHER THAN CURES?

The reason is obvious. A lifetime of prescriptions, and Big Pharma's coffers start overflowing. There is no better 'medicine' in the pharmaceutical companies' eyes than one which is highly addictive and which has to be taken for life! No wonder the pharma industry and the tobacco industry are becoming inseparable as they slice up the lucrative new e-cigarette market between themselves. Again, just look at the opioid epidemic that spread throughout the USA for supporting evidence of this exact point. It was the result of the merciless marketing of highly addictive drugs to vulnerable patients seeking pain relief.

The discovery of the Easyway method has had an incredible impact on the smoking world and helped tens of millions of prisoners to get free, but countless millions still remain in the camp, trapped by their own false beliefs and the hugely powerful influence of other nicotine addicts. On top of that are the millions of new addicts, just like you, who have been lured into nicotine addiction by vaping. You are not alone – research into the most popular Google searches for our website in the USA in 2019 indicated that – for the first time ever – the top term searched for was…

'HOW TO QUIT VAPING'

GETTING HOOKED

The influence of other vapers is what lured you into the trap in the first place. In the vast majority of cases, that first experience of nicotine will have been provided by another vaper. It seemed like a generous and flattering gesture at the time. They probably offered you your second, too, and your third. As a novice vaper you might tell yourself you won't get hooked on it, you're just dabbling. The taste and smell are odd and synthetic, so you feel confident you could never get hooked on it, but before long you're buying your own.

But the influence of other vapers doesn't stop at offering you tasters of vaping. It is mostly responsible for your own decision to start vaping and for the myths that keep you in the nicotine trap.

Ask a vaper who doesn't earn money from selling nicotine if they would recommend others to take up vaping and they are most likely to say, 'No way!' Yet unwittingly they do just that. And it's often the people who care about you most who do the most damage. Parents who smoke or vape are a powerful influence on their children. They think they can get away with the attitude of 'Do as I say, not as I do', but their lectures on the dangers of smoking or vaping are wasted if their children see them puffing away.

As a parent you might think your children will listen to the wisdom of one who knows from experience, yet all the child sees is a grown-up smoking or vaping, apparently out of choice, so of course they conclude that it must be giving them some wonderful pleasure or crutch.

The myth of pleasure or a crutch is promoted by everyone who vapes. After all, everyone knows that vaping is harmful to health, burns your money, makes you unfit and antisocial and turns you into a slave, so what other possible reason could vapers have for continuing to do it?

VAPERS DON'T ENJOY VAPING. THEY ONLY THINK THEY DO BECAUSE THEY'RE DRUG ADDICTS, AND SO THEY FEEL MOST MISERABLE WHEN THEY'RE NOT ALLOWED TO HAVE THEIR DRUG.

ALL VAPERS LIE

The trouble is, vapers convince themselves with the same Big Con. They have to because they can't live with the truth. They lie to others and they lie to themselves because the alternative is too unbearable. It's bad enough being a vaper when you block your mind to the poison, to vaper's tongue, and to the control, slavery and humiliation; if you had to face up to the grim reality day after day, life would not seem worth living.

So it suits vapers to buy into the myth because then they can pretend that there is a good reason for doing it and that they're not as helpless as it seems. Tragically, they begin to believe their own lies, as well as those of other vapers.

There are few things more pathetic than a vaper's lies. My lies as a nicotine addict were the worst! Just like them, I lied that I hadn't had nicotine when I had. They also lie about how much they vape. They lie that they can take it or leave it. They lie that they will quit.

All these lies are really an attempt to convince nobody but themselves. It is the only alternative to admitting they are pathetic, helpless slaves who get no pleasure or crutch from vaping and can't understand why they can't just quit.

LURING YOU BACK IN

You will find it useful to recognise the influence of other vapers and to harness this knowledge to help you in your own escape. All too often vapers try to scupper the efforts of those who are attempting to quit. The thought of someone escaping from the prison unnerves them because if that person succeeds, it challenges their own belief that escape is impossible and, therefore, not worth trying. As long as you have the fear of success, another vaper's escape will unsettle you. You feel like the last person left on the sinking ship.

Even when you do succeed in escaping, you will find there are always nicotine addicts ready to try and lure you back into the trap.

Make sure you are not vulnerable by preparing yourself in advance for the typical scenarios when an addict's lies might snare you.

These scenarios are very often linked to a crisis: a car crash, a bereavement, a job loss, the break-up of a relationship... when these things happen there always seems to be a smoker or vaper on hand, ready to 'comfort' you with the idea of throwing caution to the wind and having a vape.

These people aren't evil. They genuinely want to help. It's just that they don't regard you as a non-vaper but as a vaper who just happens not to be vaping at the moment. Because of the brainwashing, they assume that, like all vapers, the thing you really want at this difficult time is nicotine.

Just as vapers get youngsters hooked by offering them freebies, they do the same to adults who succumb to the temptation.

Your vaping friend is there with the supply but warns you: 'You'll get hooked again.'

'No way!' you insist. 'Maybe I'll do it just for tonight.'

But by vaping just the once you've started the cycle of addiction and soon you're back looking for more. The friends who vape are secretly pleased that you're back in the trap – it makes them feel less stupid about their own addiction.

Only a few days earlier you were a non-vaper who swore you would never buy nicotine again. Now you're having to explain to your family and friends why you couldn't last.

To begin with you protest that you only started because of a rough day, but you know the truth. You're back in the trap.

THE MIRACLE OF UNCLE JACK

When you believe that vaping provides some sort of pleasure or crutch, it's not surprising that you might feel you're helping a friend in need when you offer them a vape in a crisis. The delusion is powerful and convincing until you are shown the truth. But some of the lies that vapers and smokers tell in order to justify their decision to do it are so far-fetched it's absurd.

A classic example is the myth of Uncle Jack. Uncle Jack is a character who crops up regularly in debates about smoking – but it's the same principle as with vaping. He's a smoker who claims to have smoked 40 a day since the age of 14 and enjoyed every single one of them. Now here he is, in his 80s and still going strong. In fact, he claims never to have had a day's sickness in his life!

The implication is not just that smoking doesn't harm you, but that it's actually good for you! And there is an endless procession of people queuing up to tell you that vaping is so much safer than smoking – some even claim it is virtually risk-free.

People who argue in favour of vaping or smoking love to wheel out Uncle Jack as their star witness – living proof that all the health risks linked to nicotine addiction are not to be believed. Addicts cling doggedly to Uncle Jack to counteract the terrifying statistics society insists on throwing at us. About smoking. And increasingly about vaping.

On the evidence of one example, they are trying to build an argument against the irrefutable evidence of seven million people who die as a result of nicotine addiction each year.

Then they bring out Auntie Jane, poor dear, who never touched nicotine in her life yet died from lung cancer at the age of 50.

THE RIGHT TO VAPE

On top of this, there is the human rights argument: 'Everybody should be free to choose whether or not they take the risk of vaping.' This is the stance of the pro-nicotine movement, who use a variety of spurious arguments to try to justify their collective slavery to nicotine addiction. For example, they state that tobacco sales, JUUL sales, etc., bring in billions of pounds in taxation. So never mind the people who lose their lives and end up enslaved and impoverished as a result, it's all justified by the money!

> *VAPERS HAVE NO FREEDOM ANYWAY. THEY DO NOT*
> *CHOOSE TO GET HOOKED ANY MORE THAN A FLY*
> *CHOOSES TO GET TRAPPED BY THE PITCHER PLANT.*
> *NEITHER DO THEY CHOOSE TO REMAIN VAPERS.*

They also argue that public vaping bans lead to many vapers no longer going to bars but drinking and vaping at home instead. What's more, some argue that vapers forced outside bars so that they can vape are exposed to the risk of starting smoking as well as vaping. The notion is that when a vaper is forced outside, they may well take the attitude of: 'Oh well, I might as well smoke.' That might well be a concern if the chances of a vaper progressing to being a smoker weren't already huge. Addiction doesn't get better, it gets worse and worse, and the inclination for any addict is to get more of the drug, quicker and more efficiently… and for that reason many vapers end up lured into smoking. If you haven't fallen into the trap yet that's brilliant, and it's great that you're escaping from this addiction before reaching that stage. That said, let's not get bogged down by wondering whether at some point in the future you might have been susceptible to being lured into smoking as a result of vaping.

THE IMPORTANT THING IS THAT YOU ARE ESCAPING

It's not the vaping or smoking bans that are forcing nicotine addicts into isolation or danger; it's their addiction to nicotine, an addiction that Big Tobacco, Big Pharma, JUUL, IQOS and other pushers of nicotine work hard to maintain. Pro-nicotine groups are always funded by Big Tobacco or Big Pharma or Big Nicotine. Why do you think that is?!!

FEAR

The real motivation behind people continuing to vape or JUUL or IQOS or dip, chew, or snus is

FEAR

FEAR THAT THEY WON'T BE ABLE TO ENJOY OR COPE WITH LIFE WITHOUT NICOTINE

FEAR THAT THEY'VE GOT TO GO THROUGH SOME TERRIBLE ORDEAL TO QUIT

FEAR THAT THEY CAN NEVER BE COMPLETELY FREE FROM THE CRAVING

It doesn't dawn on them that non-nicotine addicts never suffer any of these fears or that nicotine, far from relieving their fears, causes them. The fear of success is an illusion created by a myth. Yet the fears are so great that they override the very real dangers created by nicotine addiction. As a vaper, make no mistake, the tobacco industry's involvement in vaping means only one thing: you're the victim.

ROLE MODELS

The influence of vapers on one another is reminiscent of George Orwell's *Nineteen Eighty-Four*. The creation of a society in which the people control each other through false information and fear sounds like a work of fiction, but it's something we have all witnessed in real life throughout history and it is exactly how vapers influence one another today.

In the novel *Nineteen Eighty-Four*, Big Brother, the embodiment of the system, appears to the public on 'telescreens'. Orwell was ahead of his time in recognising the influence of films and television. Hollywood and TV have played a major role in perpetuating the illusion that vaping and smoking is glamorous, cool, intellectual, interesting. The film industry has become incredibly sophisticated in finding new ways to awe our senses, but the one sense that remains detached from the action on the screen is the sense of smell.

Consequently, directors are able to portray vaping or smoking in a glamorous light, without having to deal with the reality that kissing, or even being in a room with someone, who vapes or smokes can be a foul experience, no matter how good-looking, sexy, eloquent or cool they appear to be.

On-screen heroes help to perpetuate the myths about nicotine addiction. I've already talked about the image of Sherlock Holmes smoking his pipe as he tries to think his way through the latest mysterious case. The portrayal of nicotine as an aid to concentration is commonplace in films, as is its portrayal as a social crutch, a relief for stress, a relaxation aid and a natural accompaniment for a drink, a meal and sex.

Smoking or vaping film stars are just more prisoners in the camp, but their influence is particularly strong. The power of the big screen is extraordinary. From Greta Garbo to Leonardo DiCaprio, the image of the film star with a cigarette has encouraged countless people to start smoking. During the 1970s, Hollywood woke up to the dangers of smoking and made its own attempt to cut down, with smoking appearing far less in films than it did in the days of Humphrey Bogart, James Dean and Audrey Hepburn, but today Tinseltown appears to be well and truly hooked again. In truth, it never really broke free. Whether it was Sylvester Stallone, Faye Dunaway, Steve McQueen, Clint Eastwood, John Travolta, Olivia Newton-John, Arnold Schwarzenegger, Bruce Willis, Al Pacino, Sharon Stone, Meg Ryan, Julia Roberts, Sigourney Weaver, Brad Pitt, Hugh Jackman, Uma Thurman, Scarlett Johansson, Cate Blanchett or Ryan Reynolds, they've all conspired, to a greater or lesser extent, to make cigarettes and smoking appear cool, sexy or sophisticated. Do you really think that any of them would have appeared any less desirable or cool, in any way, if they hadn't smoked? Or less tough? Or less sexy or less sophisticated? Look at the names. Remember the films.

More recently stars such as Leonardo DiCaprio, Johnny Depp, Samuel L. Jackson, Isla Fisher, Katherine Heigl, Ben Affleck, Tom Hardy and Michelle Rodriguez, to name just a few, have acted as walking, talking advertisements for vaping. This isn't by any means an exhaustive list at all. As you hear the names I have no doubt that you will be able to recall many more smoking and vaping moments in the films that you've loved throughout your life. The list spans more than 70 years.

No doubt by the time you're reading this the latest Hollywood star will have added themselves to the list. Over the years, many Hollywood stars have played a leading role in luring people into the nicotine trap and they have been paid handsomely to do so. It's not just film stars, either. TV celebrities, models, pop stars and even criminals can be powerful role models, and if they smoke their fans will smoke.

SEEING THE TRUTH TOO LATE

There are two things that make nicotine addicts stop lying. One is escaping the trap and becoming a happy non-vaper and the other is the realisation that you have inflicted physical harm on your body as a result of the addiction.

As 2020 approached a global controversy raged. On one side some public health bodies in certain countries embraced vaping wholeheartedly – without any evidence of the safety of medium- to long-term use – simply on the basis that however harmful it might be it certainly can't be as harmful as smoking. I guess if you're someone who never smoked and who then got lured into vaping, that stance is probably one that you can feel badly let down by. On the other side of the argument were health bodies who wanted to wait and see what harmful effects might result from medium- to long-term use before endorsing vaping either as a quit smoking method or as a lifestyle activity.

Whatever your experience of vaping has proved to you – whether you feel you have suffered ill effects or none whatsoever, or even if you're someone who quit smoking by vaping and now wishes to quit vaping (in which case you might consider it to have been a handy stepping stone to getting completely free) – it really doesn't matter. No part of this book is intended to use health concerns to somehow motivate you to quit. The fact is, you want to get free, and you will succeed

IN SPITE OF ANY HEALTH CONCERNS ABOUT VAPING – NOT BECAUSE OF THEM

The fact that you no longer have to concern yourself with the looming dark cloud at the back of your mind which represents the harm that vaping might, or might not, be inflicting on you, is a wonderful bonus for you to enjoy – when you are free.

You have so much to live for. It's time for you to stop being part of the Big Con. Anyone can walk free from the prison – all you have to do is ignore the influence of other vapers and nicotine addicts, see through the myths and illusions, and make your own rational decision to stop vaping once and for all.

Chapter 11

SUBSTITUTES DON'T WORK

IN THIS CHAPTER

• *THE BIG TOBACCO PROBLEM* • *DO YOU WANT TO PAY MORE TAXES?*
• *NO ILLUSIONS* • *INCREASING THE DOSE*
• *WHY WE EVEN CONSIDER SUBSTITUTES* • *BUT WHAT ABOUT DOPAMINE?*
• *NON-NICOTINE SUBSTITUTES* • *DECISION TIME*

As you prepare to have your final vape, it's time to decide what it is you really want. Are you looking for a way to keep taking nicotine without too much fear or are you looking to be free from nicotine addiction altogether?

THE BIG TOBACCO, BIG PHARMA, BIG NICOTINE PROBLEM

Over the years, the tobacco companies have invested heavily in trying to develop alternatives to cigarettes. It's easy to understand why. The industry makes staggering amounts of money from peddling a product that terrifies everybody. Imagine what it could make for a product that had the same irresistible qualities but didn't disable and kill its customers quite so quickly. Current smokers would pay even more than they spend now on cigarettes, and all those non-smokers who avoided becoming addicts because of the health risks would rush to join them.

Big Tobacco began by trying to introduce a nicotine-free cigarette. It flopped. Big Tobacco realised that in order for people to experience even the illusion of satisfaction or enjoyment the inclusion of highly addictive nicotine was essential.

Big Tobacco learned from its experiment that nicotine addiction isn't just a hazard of smoking: it is the ONLY REASON people continue to smoke. The fact that they, and Big Pharma, have used this experience to justify the use of e-cigarettes as an 'aid to quitting' is telling. If Willy Wonka had been a psychopath he would have invented a seemingly harmless, relatively calorie-light, vaping device delivering flavours like doughnut, candy floss, cupcakes and biscuits, ensuring that he also included one essential ingredient for its success…

THE MOST HIGHLY ADDICTIVE DRUG ON THE PLANET:

NICOTINE

Naturally he would've suppressed any talk of health concerns, but even if there were none…

DO YOU REALLY WANT TO SPEND THE REST OF YOUR LIFE PAYING THROUGH THE NOSE FOR THE PRIVILEGE OF BEING CONTROLLED BY A DRUG THAT CONTROLS WHAT YOU DO, WHEN YOU DO IT AND HOW YOU FEEL WHEN YOU'RE DOING IT?

It doesn't matter in what form you take nicotine – you know it's interfering with your life. That's the whole point of you following the instructions you are given in this book.

The only way of ridding yourself of this problem is to get rid of nicotine. Substitutes of any sort don't help. If they contain nicotine, that just continues the addiction and even if they don't, they create and perpetuate a feeling of unnecessary deprivation.

You don't need to replace nicotine with anything else – because nicotine was a complete hindrance to you rather than any form of pleasure or crutch. You wouldn't get rid of terrible flu and go searching for a cold to take its place.

As long as you follow the instructions throughout this book I can assure you of one thing…

*YOU WON'T MISS NICOTINE AND THEREFORE YOU WON'T
FEEL THE NEED TO REPLACE IT WITH ANYTHING*

DO YOU WANT TO PAY MORE TAXES?

In 2012/13 revenues from tobacco taxes in the UK amounted to £9.7 billion. NEARLY TEN BILLION POUNDS! Predictions that the tax yield is going to substantially decrease will, no doubt, be contradicted by the rapid emergence of JUU, IQOS and other vaping devices. The treasury departments of governments love taxable addiction for obvious reasons.

HMRC, which raises taxes on tobacco and nicotine, along with Big Tobacco, JUUL, IQOS and Big Pharma, wants you and your kids to remain lifelong nicotine addicts. You don't need any further motivation to escape from the nicotine trap, but if one were required, denying the tax departments and the pushers of nicotine your hard-earned money is a sweet one. Who wants to pay more taxes or have less disposable income?

*ONCE ESTABLISHED IN THE MARKETPLACE, THE PRICE OF
ANY ADDICTIVE PRODUCT MOVES ONLY IN ONE DIRECTION:*

UP!

This is the result of two factors:

- **The pushers want to earn more money from their captive consumer base**

- Tax policy-makers LOVE addictive products.

It all adds up to a lifetime of slavery, depriving you and your family of your happiness, freedom and wealth.

If that's how you saw JUULing or IQOSing or snusing or dipping before you'd ever tried your first experimental dose of nicotine, you wouldn't have gone near it, would you? Let alone paid for the privilege to try it out.

NO ILLUSIONS

Vapers make up all sorts of spurious reasons for why they do it. They think it looks cool, sophisticated, glamorous. They think it's sociable. They like the ritual. All these illusions go out of the window when you realise that you're doing it for one, simple, indisputable reason:

YOU'RE ADDICTED TO NICOTINE

A nicotine junkie getting their fix is no different from a heroin addict sticking a needle in their arm. Do you think heroin addicts enjoy giving themselves injections? Most people hate needles. Some faint at the sight of them. But heroin addicts can't wait for the needle to find a vein. Is that because they're anticipating a tremendous high? Or is it because they know that the panic and misery they're suffering is about to be relieved? The fact is, they no longer know the difference.

Watch the reaction of a heroin addict as the drug enters their blood-stream. It's not pleasure; it's relief, like the relief of taking off tight shoes. It's not the beginning of something good; it's the ending of something bad – albeit for just a short time. It's the thief giving his victim £10 back from the £100 he stole, and the victim being fooled into gratitude.

Heroin addicts don't enjoy the needle going into their arm. That's just the way they get their drug. Without going into graphic detail, the process of finding a vein anywhere in their body becomes a truly humiliating, shameful and degrading process for the addict. There are clear similarities between all drug addictions. However, there is one key difference: heroin addicts know they only inject themselves to get the heroin, whereas nicotine addicts believe they vape because they enjoy vaping for its own sake. The same goes for all nicotine addiction.

The way nicotine traps its victims is much more subtle than the way heroin traps the heroin addict. Nicotine addicts think they enjoy it because it appears to relieve the empty, insecure feeling that they perceive to be part of normal life. Non-nicotine addicts don't suffer it and neither did you before you took your first experimental doses of nicotine. But because of the gradual decline that they experience, vapers regard the empty, insecure feeling of nicotine withdrawal as 'normal'. As they slide further into the trap they continually adjust their perception of 'normal', not realising that they're slipping way below a genuinely normal, healthy level of wellbeing, one which is not subject to the albeit mild discomfort of virtually constant withdrawal.

When you quit, you will be amazed at how far below a genuine level of normality you had been, because of vaping. Without the panic of nicotine addiction, you will feel more relaxed, confident, happy and healthy ALL THE TIME.

A couple of centuries ago, nicotine addicts got their fix by sniffing dust up their nose in the form of snuff. In the Wild West and on the baseball pitch, they stuck a plug of tobacco between their cheek and gum and continually spat out the repulsive juice. If you've ever tried chewing tobacco and made the mistake of swallowing, you'll understand the need to keep spitting. The taste is pure poison.

Be under no illusions. Whether you sniff snuff, chew tobacco, smoke cigarettes, use snus, suck nicotine sticks, chew nicotine gum, stick a patch on your skin, or vape, the methods of taking nicotine have nothing to do with pleasure. It's all about getting the drug into your bloodstream in an effort to gain some kind of relief from nicotine withdrawal (the Little Monster) and the nagging mental battle (the Big Monster).

INCREASING THE DOSE

The natural tendency with drug addiction is to take more and more of the drug. This is the result of the body building up tolerance to poison – you end up needing more of the drug to have an equal effect.

Big Tobacco, Big Pharma and Big Nicotine have pumped hundreds of millions of dollars into producing a variety of different devices that have one simple function:

TO GET YOU ADDICTED AND KEEP YOU ADDICTED

FOR THE REST OF YOUR LIFE

The industry doesn't just want *you*.

IT WANTS YOUR BROTHERS AND SISTERS

IT WANTS YOUR FRIENDS

IT WANTS YOUR KIDS

FOR THE REST OF THEIR LIVES

You don't need me to sell you the idea of the joy of being free – that's the desire which compelled you to pick up this book. It's just that at the moment you're not sure you can get free and even less sure that you can stay free. You have been convinced that even if you do get free, and stay free, it's going to be a battle for the rest of your life.

I only have good news for you. You can look forward to finishing this book, walking to freedom and enjoying every single moment of it as if you'd never been lured into trying those first experimental shots of nicotine. All you have to do is go on reading while carrying on using nicotine in whatever form you use it, and follow the instructions.

WHY WE EVEN CONSIDER SUBSTITUTES

Some are tempted to use substitutes in an attempt to get free from one form of nicotine delivery system by adopting another. Some resort to using nicotine gum in an attempt to get free from JUUL or IQOS or other devices. Some long-term gum chewers attempt to get free by switching to e-cigarettes or patches or other nicotine-delivering products. Once you understand addiction, you can see the pointlessness of attempting to do so.

One of the main arguments put forward by some members of the medical profession and tobacco control establishment (when promoting nicotine products which aren't burned) is that nicotine is a relatively harmless drug. Tell that to the hundreds of millions of poor nicotine addicts that it's slaughtered over the years. Aside from that, if you were happy to remain a nicotine addict for the rest of your life, they might have a point. But isn't your reason for reading this book to get free from being controlled by nicotine? As I said right at the beginning – it really doesn't matter whether the health concerns surrounding JUUL, IQOS or any other nicotine delivery device are overstated by some or understated by others.

WHETHER THE HEALTH CONCERNS WORRY YOU OR NOT – IT REALLY DOESN'T MATTER

Focusing on them either way will cause you a problem in the future as the argument about levels of harm rages on from one extreme to the other.

DON'T MAKE THEM A MOTIVATION FOR FREEDOM

Instead, appreciate the freedom of not having to even consider them any more. It's a wonderful bonus when you are free.

Using nicotine substitutes doesn't work as a cure for nicotine addiction because it is based on three false beliefs:

- that the physical withdrawal is painful

- that vaping, JUULing, IQOSing, chewing, dipping or snusing is a habit

• that people don't mind being addicted.

But the real truth is that:

• the physical withdrawal from nicotine is virtually imperceptible

• nicotine addiction is not a habit – it's drug addiction

• no one wants to be addicted to anything.

The fabulous thing about understanding the addiction is that, although highly effective in hooking its victims, the addiction itself is actually extremely weak and easy to break free from... as long as you know how.

For anyone who still believes that vaping gives them some sort of benefit or crutch, cutting down gradually is a real struggle. It goes against everything their mind and body are crying out for. As you've learned already, the nicotine trap takes you on a downward spiral because each dose of nicotine never fully satisfies the craving created by the one before, so you are always wanting to increase the dose.

THE TENDENCY WITH ALL DRUGS IS TO TAKE MORE, NOT LESS

Now let's focus on a really important issue. Ask yourself a question:

WHAT'S SO GREAT ABOUT BEING A VAPER (OR USER OF NICOTINE IN ANY FORM)?

It's possible that you've never really reflected on this in much detail before. There must be a word to describe the feeling you get when you vape, surely?

WHAT'S THE WORD?

The English language is a rich, deep, varied language that has evolved over many centuries. Let's use that fact to probe further into understanding the so-called pleasure of nicotine.

If you were to drink alcohol there is a word, actually there are many, to describe the effect, the perceived pleasure, of doing so. Words such as 'tipsy, merry, sloshed or inebriated' – there are many, many more.

• Someone who takes heroin would say they get 'smacked up'.

• Someone who takes cocaine might be 'wired' or 'coked up'.

• Someone who takes MDMA or ecstasy might claim to feel 'loved up'.

• Users of cannabis would say they're 'stoned' or 'high' or 'baked' or 'blazed'.

So bearing all that in mind – what is the unique word or phrase to describe the pleasure or the high that you achieve from vaping, JUULing, IQOSing, nicotine gum, dip, snus or any other nicotine product? Remember, we're not talking about the products that contain cannabis and a whole host of other mind-altering drugs here – we're talking about nicotine.

Did you ever overhear someone at a party bragging about being 'Really nicotined up' or 'I'm totally nicotined'? Of course you haven't. You may well have come across someone who was feeling lousy because they'd had too much nicotine.

Think about how long smoking has been around for, compared to vaping; hundreds of years – yet the English language has failed to adopt a word that describes the perceived pleasure of the drug.

Some smokers and vapers who attend our seminars say they get 'a buzz or a high' from their first cigarette or vape after a long period of not having had one. Yet that isn't a buzz or a high – it's simply 'dizzy'. It's caused by the poison going into your body and brain – you can get exactly the same sensation by holding your breath for 30 seconds or spinning around while you count to 10. Don't do it – it isn't much fun and you'll make yourself feel lousy. It's certainly not a high.

So bearing all that in mind – what is the unique word or phrase to describe the pleasure or the high that you achieve from smoking a cigarette or JUULing or IQOSing or taking nicotine in any form?

THERE ISN'T ONE!

The English language is a rich and diverse language, a language that provides us with 14 words for rain, yet there is not one unique word in the entire English language which describes the pleasure obtained from nicotine. Why not?

BECAUSE IT DOESN'T EXIST

It's perfectly natural to have doubts. But bear in mind that the English language does not have any doubts at all.

EVEN IF IT'S ILLUSORY – SURELY FEELING BETTER WHEN YOU HAVE A VAPE IS LIKE A BOOST? DOES IT REALLY MATTER IF IT ISN'T REAL?

EXERCISE: GAINING AN ILLUSORY BOOST

Let's try a quick exercise to cover this question. Put your hands in the air. As high as you can go so it's a little uncomfortable. Now I'd like you to consider two options and please consider both before making your decision regarding which one to take.

Option One: you are welcome to put your hands straight down

Option Two: you can keep your hands up for the next 15 minutes and then put them down again, therefore obtaining the wonderful illusory pleasure of doing so.

Make your mind up now please – you can either put them straight back down or keep them up for 15 minutes.

If you're dismissing this exercise and maintaining that at least an illusory boost is better than no boost at all, then please ensure that you keep your hands up high, so it's a little uncomfortable, for a further 14½ minutes before proceeding with this book.

Of course, there's no point in putting your hands up for 15 minutes for the sake of putting them down... it would be like wearing tight shoes just for the relief of taking them off. Painful and pointless.

BUT WHAT ABOUT DOPAMINE?

Vapers use all kinds of excuses and reasoning to justify their continued vaping or JUULing. In a desperate attempt to explain their continued addiction (and failure to quit) they seek solace in scientific explanations of what it is they might enjoy about nicotine. These often involve talk of nicotine raising dopamine levels.

Please don't be deterred by some of the complex wording that follows – to quit vaping easily you don't need to understand the workings of brain function with regard to nicotine addiction, any more than you need to understand the complex workings of the internal combustion engine to learn to drive a car. Look at the road, not under the bonnet; let the method work for you and you'll be a happy non-vaper and non-nicotine addict in no time at all.

Some people claim that nicotine helps with depression and anxiety, but if this were true then surely all nicotine addicts would be less anxious and less depressed than non-addicts? Yet research shows the exact opposite – that they are much more anxious and more depressed than non-addicts.

Tragically there's no doubt that a good portion of people who live with depression and anxiety are drawn into nicotine addiction by the flawed belief that nicotine might help them handle their condition – that's all part of the brainwashing.

Humans are programmed to seek out dopamine-elevating activities to ensure good health, happiness and longevity/survival. Examples are making love, eating, listening to music, hugging children, animals or a partner or a friend, socialising and exercising. These are natural, normal, healthy activities and behaviours that a normal, uncorrupted, functioning 'reward system' is designed to reinforce.

Back when nicotine addiction was at its peak in the form of smoking, we didn't know how nicotine and other drugs affected the brain. Since then we have learned a great deal about a function of the brain known colloquially as reward pathways.

*In the brain dopamine functions as a neurotransmitter –
a chemical released by neurons (nerve cells) to send
signals to other nerve cells. The reward pathways
play a major role in the motivational component of
reward-motivated, or reinforced, behaviour.*

Can you imagine the disruption that can be caused to this natural, instinctive process by the introduction of a highly addictive drug, one which appears to relieve the discomfort created by the first dose, and every subsequent dose?

It's of tremendous comfort to everyone working within Easyway, who for decades have been working tirelessly to cure addiction all over the world, that as more and more becomes known about the way nicotine influences dopamine, science confirms what Allen Carr's Easyway has been asserting for more than 35 years.

In 2019, Professor Robert West, one of the world's leading academics in the field of nicotine addiction, stated publicly:

*"Nicotine causes dopamine release by nerve cells that
make up the 'reward system' in the brain, including the
nucleus accumbens – a part of the brain involved in learning
to do things. The dopamine release tells the brain to pay
attention to the situation and what the smoker was just
doing – and do the same thing next time they're in that same
situation. So, a link is forged between the impulse to smoke
and situations in which smoking normally happens."*

Importantly, Professor West went on to add:

Crucially, the smoker doesn't have to feel any
pleasure or enjoyment for this to work.

A smoker or vaper's first experience of nicotine is normally at worst extremely unpleasant and at best a little unpleasant or ambivalent. For the sake of understanding this, addicts have to ignore the feelings aroused by the circumstances surrounding their first experience of nicotine; the peer pressure and praise, the feeling of rebelliousness, the feeling of fitting in, the sense of appearing stylish, sophisticated or macho. None of those are caused by the introduction of nicotine to the body, they're all to do with the environment and the company in which the nicotine is taken.

So most nicotine addicts remember the physical effect of their first dose of nicotine as being unpleasant or ambivalent and this alone disproves any notion that nicotine's initial introduction to the body and brain caused huge feelings of 'pleasure'. Whatever impact nicotine has on dopamine levels when first introduced to the body, it's certainly not pleasurable. In fact, in the case of smoking, most people's first cigarette is so unpleasant and unrewarding it convinces them that they could never become addicted. The reason smokers and vapers develop a deep-seated belief that it IS pleasurable is explained by Professor West perfectly.

POINT A: NICOTINE WITHDRAWAL IS THE RESULT OF THE FIRST EVER DOSE OF NICOTINE THE ADDICT TOOK.

The withdrawal is momentarily 'relieved' by the next dose of nicotine. The brain concludes, non-consciously: 'Next time you feel nicotine withdrawal – do that again!' In other words, the behaviour of having a vape in response to experiencing nicotine withdrawal is reinforced every time a vaper vapes regardless of the fact that the next vape will also cause nicotine withdrawal.

Whether a vaper is in a happy situation, a concentration situation, a sad situation, a stress situation, a relaxing situation, a boring situation or a lonely situation, they simultaneously experience nicotine withdrawal, and respond by having a vape. The withdrawal is partially relieved and they immediately feel better than a moment before. Yet they are oblivious to the fact that the vape did nothing except partially relieve the withdrawal. It is in this way that the nicotine addict is fooled into believing that vaping helps at these times. They don't realise that the vape perpetuates nicotine withdrawal – it doesn't relieve it.

It's no wonder nicotine addicts think nicotine not only helps them to be happy or cope with sadness and stress but also helps them concentrate, relax or cope with boredom or loneliness! It's got nothing to do with *genuine* pleasure or *genuine* improvement of mood. And every single time they vape in one of those situations the brain concludes, non-consciously: 'Next time that happens – do that again!'

Non-nicotine addicts don't have to deal with any of the mental and physical aggravation of being addicted to nicotine. They don't suffer nicotine poisoning, nicotine withdrawal or the aberrational/unnatural impact nicotine has on dopamine and their behaviour.

POINT B: ALL A VAPER IS TRYING TO ACHIEVE WHEN THEY VAPE IS TO RECAPTURE THE FEELING OF PEACE, CALM, TRANQUILLITY AND COMPLETENESS THEY ENJOYED THEIR ENTIRE LIFE BEFORE THEY HAD THEIR FIRST EXPERIMENTAL VAPE.

In other words – a vaper vapes in order to feel like a non-vaper.

Once a nicotine addict understands Point A and Point B, we can explain how nicotine addiction, irrespective of nicotine's influence on dopamine levels, is actually extremely mild, and that the really unpleasant symptoms any addict suffers when they try to quit without Easyway's help are the result of a mental struggle. That struggle is caused by the nicotine addict feeling deprived of what they think is a genuine pleasure or crutch.

The contents of this book are designed to reveal how the nicotine addict's belief system surrounding their drug – that it helps them to relax, socialise, handle stress, concentrate, enjoy alcohol, take a break from work, and so on – is illusory. All of it is based on misinformation, misinterpretation of personal experiences and their addiction to nicotine.

The addict then concludes that there aren't any factual advantages or benefits to be obtained from vaping and therefore there is no point in doing it. This effectively destroys the belief that they are dependent on the drug and simultaneously removes the desire to vape, therefore neutralising the addiction.

ALLEN CARR'S EASYWAY REWIRES YOUR BRAIN

This leaves the addict to handle the extremely mild symptoms of nicotine withdrawal without having to experience the discomfort of feeling that they are missing out on something they used to enjoy or receive benefit from.

This is hugely important, as the former addict develops new responses to any habitual triggers to vape over the first few weeks of being a happy non-addict. For example, if they used to vape as they left work in the afternoon, that might be a moment when the thought of vaping crosses their mind, but once they quit with Easyway, instead of consciously processing thoughts and feelings of loss, they process thoughts and feelings of release and freedom.

This is not a case of mind over matter or simple positive thinking – it's a case of seeing things as they really are.

I was once told about an ancient tribe who believe that if you draw a chalk circle around them, they are unable to move outside of it. There's no physical barrier – but their belief is enough to make them remain captive. The same can be said of the nicotine addict's beliefs in support of their continued addiction. Correcting those beliefs is the key to getting free and staying free and, more importantly, doing so while feeling fabulous.

NON-NICOTINE SUBSTITUTES

Anything that you use as a substitute for vaping perpetuates the illusion that you're making a sacrifice when you quit.

Sweets, chocolate and normal chewing gum are common substitutes used by nicotine addicts trying to quit. Whenever they feel the nicotine craving, they have a sweet, a chocolate or a piece of gum instead of vaping. This is only moving the problem, not solving it. The empty, insecure feeling of the body withdrawing from nicotine feels the same as hunger, but food does not relieve it. It might take your mind off the craving for a little while, but it doesn't remove the feeling of sacrifice. As long as the Big Monster is still alive in your brain, you will never be free from the desire to vape. You won't need any kind of substitute after you quit and using one, even one that doesn't contain nicotine, will cause you to fail. It will create, and perpetuate, an unnecessary feeling of deprivation.

DECISION TIME

So it's time to decide what you really want. All nicotine addicts dream of a substitute that gives them the feeling of relaxation they get when they vape, without any of the disadvantages – health concerns, the cost, slavery and stigma.

GOOD NEWS!

This is exactly what you get when you quit vaping and get free from nicotine.

That feeling of relaxation is what non-nicotine addicts have all the time. It is merely the feeling of relief from nicotine craving. Non-addicts don't suffer from nicotine craving.

THE ONLY REASON YOU VAPE IS TO FEEL LIKE A NON-VAPER FEELS ALL THE TIME

In order to become a happy non-vaper, you do need to conquer two enemies, but habit has nothing to do with it and you won't suffer any pain. One of those enemies is the Little Monster in your body, which feeds on nicotine and cries out when it's hungry. The cries of the Little Monster are so slight as to be almost imperceptible. You don't need a gradual weaning process to cope with the physical sensation of withdrawal.

The only threat from the Little Monster is that it wakes up the Big Monster in your brain, which interprets the Little Monster's cries as 'I want a vape'. The Big Monster makes you fixate on having a vape and causes you to feel deprived and miserable if you can't. Continue to feed the Little Monster and you prolong the life of both of your enemies.

Chapter 12

ARE YOU WORRIED ABOUT YOUR WEIGHT?

IN THIS CHAPTER
• *CONFLICTING EVIDENCE* • *HUNGER VS NICOTINE WITHDRAWAL*
• *WHY SOME SMOKERS AND VAPERS LOSE WEIGHT* • *WHAT IS HUNGER?*
• *BLINDED BY SCIENCE* • *ACHIEVING YOUR IDEAL WEIGHT*
• *THE FINAL PROOF*

You may be aware of the theory that vaping helps to keep your weight down, which may cause you to worry that you will gain weight if you quit. There is actually no need to worry at all. The effect of vaping on weight is a myth. Easyway will show you how to quit without putting on any weight at all. I want to take a few moments to elaborate on this important issue.

CONFLICTING EVIDENCE

The myth that vaping, or for that matter smoking, keeps you thin is based on the evidence of people who try to quit with the willpower method and find themselves putting on weight. Naturally, they assume that the vape or cigarettes were keeping them thin. There are plenty of people like this about and remember, people who quit with the willpower method love to let everyone know all about their unbearable struggle.

We hear a lot less from those who quit without any problem. There are enough examples of people who lose weight after quitting to cast considerable doubt on any theory that vaping or smoking keeps you thin. There are also plenty of overweight vapers and smokers who'll be scratching their heads at this theory.

I used to joke, 'I'm not overweight, I'm just six inches shorter than I should be' during my years as a heavy smoker. As a nicotine addict I was two stone overweight even though I was a virtual chain smoker.

Smoking did not make me thin, yet whenever I tried to quit I somehow gained more weight... with one notable exception. When I stopped smoking and escaped nicotine addiction for good, I lost two stone within six months of becoming nicotine-free.

So what are we supposed to believe? Does vaping or smoking make you put on weight or does it keep your weight down? Let's unravel the myth and see the true picture.

HUNGER VS NICOTINE WITHDRAWAL

Previously I've mentioned that the empty, insecure feeling of nicotine withdrawing from the body feels the same as hunger. It's a feeling which is so slight that it rarely captures your attention but it does trigger automatic responses. With hunger, your body is asking you to respond by feeding it with food; with nicotine withdrawal, the Little Monster is demanding you feed it with nicotine.

The feelings are the same, their sources are very different. One is a natural survival instinct, the other is drug addiction. And, most importantly, you can't satisfy the cravings by substituting nicotine for food or vice versa.

VAPING WILL NOT SATISFY HUNGER

FOOD WILL NOT STOP NICOTINE CRAVINGS

If your car is overheating, it could be because the engine is low on oil or because the cooling system is low on water. If you top up the oil with water or top up the coolant with oil, you won't fix the problem. In fact, you'll destroy the machine!

People who try to quit with the willpower method try to satisfy the craving, or take their mind off it, by treating it as if it was hunger. They substitute vaping with junk food. Chewing gum and sweets are the common choice. Of course, they don't even satisfy hunger, let alone nicotine craving. So you move on to more substantial foods in your efforts to satisfy what feels like a permanent hunger.

The willpower method perpetuates the myth that you're making a sacrifice, so when you quit with willpower your body and brain are always expecting little rewards. If you regard cakes, biscuits and chocolate bars as rewards, or burgers, fries and other junk foods, you will eat to excess in an attempt to overcome the feeling of deprivation.

This is why people who quit with the willpower method put on weight. But because of the myth that vaping or smoking keeps your weight down, you assume the weight gain is due to 'giving up' nicotine.

When you quit with Easyway, you don't feel like you're 'giving up' anything; only making wonderful gains. There's no psychological need for extra rewards.

WHY SOME SMOKERS AND VAPERS LOSE WEIGHT

The confusion between hunger and nicotine craving also explains why some smokers and vapers do get thinner. Instead of eating when hungry, they vape or smoke. First thing in the morning, when you wake up, both vapers and non-vapers instinctively relieve a number of needs. We relieve our bladders, we relieve our thirst and non-vapers also relieve their hunger. Vapers, however, are more likely to fire up their vaping device.

As the hunger intensifies, the vaper continues to confuse the need with their craving for nicotine, so they vape more. Most long-term vapers, however, have the opposite problem. They eat when they feel the craving for nicotine. Of course, eating doesn't satisfy the Little Monster. Neither does vaping – not fully. Because of your tolerance to the poison, you go through life with what feels like a permanent hunger. The tendency is to try and satisfy this feeling by eating as well as vaping.

When opportunities to vape are restricted, vapers will eat instead. This isn't a conscious choice; they are instinctively responding to a sensation that feels just like hunger. If they could vape they would, but without being able to vape they reach for the next available option.

If vaping actually helped you to keep your weight down, you would expect most heavy vapers to be slim. In fact, most heavy vapers are overweight.

WHAT IS HUNGER?

Hunger is a crucial and ingenious part of your body's survival toolkit, which we talked about earlier. It works rather like the fuel gauge on your car. When your body is running low on the vital nutrients it needs, it sends a signal to your brain that feels like an emptiness in your stomach, and your brain responds by looking for things to eat.

When your car's fuel gauge approaches empty, what do you do? Drive to the nearest lake or river and fill up with water? Drive to a builder's yard and fill up with sand? Of course not, you pull in at the next petrol station and fill up with the right type of fuel.

Your body is just as specific about the fuel it needs. When it signals hunger, it's not asking for any old rubbish to be forced into your digestive system; it's asking for the specific vitamins, minerals, fibre, protein, carbohydrates, etc., which your body needs to stay healthy and strong. Respond to hunger by filling up with junk food and you won't satisfy that need; therefore you will not satisfy your hunger, and so you will keep eating and put on weight.

You can find out more about hunger and sugar and carb addiction with *Allen Carr's Good Sugar Bad Sugar: Eat yourself free from sugar and carb addiction.*

BLINDED BY SCIENCE

Like most of the vaping myths, the one about vaping keeping you thin is reinforced by certain 'so-called' experts, who have added a couple of scientific twists to the theory. One is that vaping speeds up your metabolism, which means you burn off fat faster.

If this was the case, how do they explain why most heavy vapers and smokers are overweight and why vapers and smokers who quit with Easyway tend to lose weight after they quit? Surely, if their metabolism slowed down they would put on weight?

Another theory is that vaping and smoking are appetite suppressants. In other words, they reduce your desire for food. This theory is based on three facts:

1. Many vapers who quit eat more and put on weight. This is because when nicotine addicts quit with the willpower method they feel deprived and try to substitute nicotine by eating and drinking more.

2. The confusion between nicotine craving and hunger fools

nicotine addicts into thinking they're hungry when they're craving nicotine and if they vape in that moment, the partial relief of the nicotine craving fools them into thinking the vaping has relieved their hunger.

3. Hunger pangs come and go. Non-vapers know they don't have to eat every time they feel a hunger pang. It's a very mild sensation and it will subside after a short time if they ignore it. However, if a vaper feels a hunger pang and vapes, they credit the vape when the pang subsides. In fact, the pang would have subsided anyway. They have no idea this is what happens to non-vapers all the time.

You can always find a 'so-called' expert coming up with complicated theories when the truth is staring us all in the face.

YOU WILL PUT ON WEIGHT WHEN YOU STOP VAPING IF YOU START SUBSTITUTING FOOD FOR NICOTINE

But when you use Easyway, that doesn't happen. When you quit, the Little Monster will continue to cry out for its fix for a few days. The feeling is so slight as to be almost imperceptible, but if you think you're making a sacrifice it will make you feel deprived and miserable. With this method you have your final shot of nicotine knowing that you're not sacrificing anything. On the contrary, you're making marvellous gains. So you can rejoice in the death throes of the Little Monster without feeling any need for substitutes. Find that hard to believe? Just you wait and see.

ACHIEVING YOUR IDEAL WEIGHT

There are two factors that determine whether you lose or gain weight. One is diet; the other is exercise. If you take in more fuel than you burn off, you will gain weight. Burn off more than you take in and you will lose weight.

There are factors that influence the amount you consume and the amount you burn, and vaping is one of them. The confusion between hunger and nicotine craving makes some vapers eat more and others eat less. Nicotine and other poisons contained in vaping create an underlying feeling of lethargy, which can be as subtle as just feeling constantly a little out of sorts.

One of the marvellous gains you can look forward to is feeling more vital and more energetic. A key instruction with Easyway is not to alter your lifestyle just because you have quit vaping. I will explain why later. But when you quit, you may well feel more inclined to take regular exercise because you've got the energy and confidence for it. Exercise gets the adrenaline flowing and makes you feel great. It's the best stimulant there is – a genuine high!

If you're out of condition, start slowly and don't push yourself too hard. There's no need. You've got the rest of your life.

Once you've solved your nicotine problem, you'll have so much more confidence and energy that you'll be far better equipped to solve other problems, such as weight.

If you've been relying on vaping to keep your weight down, you can abandon that policy now. Any success you've had in keeping your weight down is in spite of being a nicotine addict, not because of it. Believe that nicotine gives you any kind of benefit and you're more likely to put on weight, either by remaining an addict and feeling confused or by quitting and feeling deprived and substituting food and drink for the vaping.

THE FINAL PROOF

If you're still not convinced that the 'so-called' experts have got it wrong, ask yourself this: why is there no such thing as The Diet Vape? Imagine if Big Tobacco or Big Pharma had conclusive proof that vaping kept your weight down; don't you think they would shout about it from the rooftops and bring out a brand specifically aimed at dieters? So why haven't they? Quite simply because:

VAPING DOES NOT HELP YOU LOSE WEIGHT

If it did, the manufacturers would say so. No one could stop them. Instead they use celebrity promotions and product placement to imply it! It's phoney! Don't swallow their lies any more.

Actually, I have no doubt that within a couple of years Big Tobacco will have somehow harnessed the illusion that vaping helps addicts control their weight. That would enable them to make bold, and baseless, claims that nicotine can help people keep slim. Such is the power and influence of this multi-billion-dollar addiction racket. After all, this is an industry which has repeatedly lied, even under oath, and suppressed evidence of harm and addiction over decades, while killing more than half of their customers 10, 20 or 30 years before their time. Their power and influence is growing rather than shrinking, though. You only have to look at Philip Morris International's obscene attempts to infiltrate the anti-tobacco establishment by claiming that they are the solution to the developed world's smoking problem rather than THE problem... while continuing to aggressively market cigarettes to kids in other parts of the world. They are blatant, dangerous hypocrites.

And it's not just Big Tobacco that is the problem – even though it has a tight hold on the tobacco AND vaping industry.

THE RISE AND RISE OF JUUL

Just a quick look at a company like JUUL tells you all you need to know.

Adam Bowen and James Monsees co-founded JUUL Labs with (apparently) the intention of providing a safer alternative source of nicotine for smokers. On paper, the principle of harm-reduction has good arguments, as well as some downsides.

Yet in spite of JUUL's apparently philanthropic objectives they proceeded to market, advertise and push their highly addictive product to kids. In 2018 and 2019 the first evidence of a merciless, savage policy of funding campaigns that deliberately targeted kids emerged. JUUL had gone from being a start-up to a behemoth corporation valued at more than...

$38 BILLION

In just a few short years. That's quite a start-up!

Following the launch of investigations by the US Federal Trade Commission, the US Food & Drug Administration and a host of State Attorney Generals into JUUL's targeting of youngsters – and the restrictive legislation designed to protect kids from JUUL's influence that is likely to result – the value of the company sank to $24 BILLION.

The appointment of key executives from Big Tobacco will no doubt help them navigate through the impending legislation and avoid or minimise any financial penalties and obligations. This will allow them to rebuild the company's value, no doubt finding ways to continue to market their products to kids. In any event – they will probably be replaced by the next 'new, exciting, young' brand that Big Tobacco devises or acquires and puts into play.

IT'S EASY WHEN YOU KNOW HOW.
AND BIG TOBACCO KNOWS HOW.

What did I say earlier?

IF WILLY WONKA HAD BEEN A PSYCHOPATH...

Not giving your hard-earned money to people like this is a wonderful bonus which will be obtained as a result of your freedom.

Chapter 13

THE ADVANTAGES OF VAPING

Chapter 14

ALL VAPERS ARE THE SAME

IN THIS CHAPTER

•WOMEN VAPERS •RESTRICTING YOUR VAPING
•A WORD TO THE WISE ABOUT CANNABIS/THC •OCCASIONAL VAPERS
•STOPPERS AND STARTERS •THE SECRET VAPER

The addictive personality myth feeds the belief that some vapers are more susceptible to the nicotine trap than others and some can control their intake of nicotine better than others. So let's try to identify which type of nicotine addict you are and which type you would really like to be.

WOMEN VAPERS

Tobacco companies don't claim that cigarettes keep you slim because they can't – it's not true. Advertising, for all its vices, still has to carry at least a modicum of truth. All they can do is perpetuate the myth by putting their products in the hands of slender film stars, models and other female icons. Sadly, the marketing works.

The 'free pass' that some vaping companies are getting from the health authorities in various countries will, no doubt, lead to a host of highly questionable scientific studies designed to prove that vaping helps with weight control. Be wary of these. It's the same machine trying to do the same job.

The key is seeing through the illusions and understanding the true picture: that vaping does not relieve stress or provide any kind of crutch at all; neither does it suppress your appetite or help you stay slim.

The truth is...

NICOTINE DOES NOTHING FOR YOU WHATSOEVER

RESTRICTING YOUR VAPING

Think about this carefully. When it comes to deciding what type of vaper or nicotine addict you want to be, there are two questions you should ask yourself:

1. **How much would you vape if you could choose your ideal amount?**

Having decided how often you would like to vape, the next question is:

2. **Why don't you vape that much now?**

No one forces you to vape, or snus or chew tobacco or nicotine gum. It is only you who takes the nicotine from the pack. If you want to do it less often, who's stopping you?

Vapers envy anyone who does it less than them because they think they're getting the best of both worlds: they're getting their pleasure or crutch and they don't appear to be enslaved by vaping. In short, they appear to be in control.

In fact, both beliefs are false. There is no pleasure or crutch from vaping or any form of nicotine and light vapers suffer just as much in the nicotine trap as heavy ones. In fact, they suffer more because they are constantly fighting the urge to do it more.

Any vaper who has tried to cut down knows that restricting the amount you vape through willpower will only work for a limited period at best.

When your vaping is restricted by factors such as bans in public places, it's easy to go without because there is no question of doing it. Just like the student in the exam, when you know that vaping is not an option, the Big Monster doesn't bother you. It's only when you can vape but try to stop yourself from doing so that the Big Monster begins to torment you.

Some ex-vapers fall into the trap again because they grow overconfident and think they can have 'just the occasional vape' without getting hooked. They still believe they have made a sacrifice, they think they deserve a reward and they think they can control their vaping. It's the same delusion that leads them to get hooked in the first place. Even if you think you have many strong reasons for vaping, you wouldn't have that one puff if you knew you would have to continue doing it for the rest of your life.

DAY IN

DAY OUT

EVERY SINGLE DAY

FOR THE REST OF YOUR LIFE

NEVER BEING ALLOWED TO STOP

Be very clear about this:

THERE IS NO SUCH THING AS 'JUST ONE PUFF'

If you vape on one occasion, what's to stop you doing it again? And again? And again?

THERE IS ALWAYS ANOTHER AND ANOTHER AND ANOTHER

A WORD TO THE WISE ABOUT CANNABIS/THC

Apologies to anyone reading this who has never and would never touch illicit drugs under any circumstances. That said, it is an issue that we need to cover, purely because it's an issue that arises for many, many vapers.

At our centres around the world, we're often (rather sheepishly) asked by clients whether they have to stop smoking or vaping cannabis. To be clear, we don't encourage, endorse or recommend the use of any illicit drug, but as long as the smoker avoids mixing their drug with nicotine they're perfectly able to carry on using it as long as they don't vape it.

There are proven links between cannabis vape and deaths from vaping, but aside from those, it's virtually impossible to guarantee that any vape ingredients are nicotine-free.

There are huge question marks over the safety of vaping with or without THC. As I said earlier, health concerns aren't a great motivating factor, but release from them IS a wonderful bonus to enjoy when you get free. The crux of the issue with cannabis or THC (or whatever) is why take such a foolish risk by vaping it? There are lots of less risky ways of imbibing the drug (although they are still not risk-free). Don't misunderstand me, we're not saying taking anything like that is a good idea – what we are saying is if you do take it then make sure you use the least dangerous means.

When you quit vaping you don't have to stop using those drugs, but you do need to stop vaping them.

YOU CANNOT DO THIS WITH THC AND OTHER ILLICIT DRUG PRODUCTS DESIGNED FOR VAPING, but we give the following advice to smokers at our centres who smoke weed mixed with tobacco. Those who want to quit nicotine but don't want to quit weed are recommended to use a pipe or a bowl or to hot-knife it – in other words, have it neat – instead of mixing it with tobacco.

There are three important caveats to this advice:

• It would be far better, from a health point of view, to find a less toxic way of taking the drug – in tea, for example.

• Never, ever let the fact that you 'get away' with having neat joints encourage you to be so confident of your freedom that, at some point in the future, you casually share a joint containing tobacco at a social event. If you do, you'll be hooked on nicotine again in no time at all. GUARANTEED! Don't do it!

• Don't use joints as substitutes. If you attempt to replace cigarettes or vaping with neat joints, you'll lose your job, your partner, your house and your whole purpose in life, seemingly without a care in the world! My tongue is firmly in my cheek on this point, but please don't let that detract from this warning

– any substitute, of any sort, let alone one containing one of the drugs mentioned, will lead you straight back to nicotine addiction again.

I repeat –

YOU CANNOT USE THC AND OTHER ILLICIT DRUG PRODUCTS DESIGNED FOR VAPING IN A NEAT FORM

Who knows what the dangers of vaping really are? What are the odds that it might cause irreparable harm? When it comes to nicotine addiction most vapers tell themselves that any harmful effects will never happen to them. They're burying their head in the sand.

It's amazing how a vaper will buy, for example, a lottery ticket in the hope that they will win. Now, in the EuroMillions Lottery, the chances of winning the jackpot are one in 140 million.

ONE CHANCE IN ONE HUNDRED AND FORTY MILLION!

Why do they buy a ticket? The thought process is:

'SOMEONE'S GOT TO WIN IT – IT COULD BE ME!'

Yet whatever risks a vaper might consider will be dismissed. What do they think?

'IT WON'T BE ME!'

Think about it. A one in 140 million chance of being a multi-millionaire and we'll not only buy a ticket but keep our fingers crossed. Then we'll check the result with a sense of excitement, expectation and hope.

Yet whatever risk there is from vaping – we dismiss it.

'IT WON'T BE ME!'

Can you see the anomaly here?

I'm telling you this not to worry you, and certainly not to scare you. I just want to ensure that you are beginning to see the nicotine trap for what it is, and are looking forward to all the amazing, fantastic bonuses you're set to enjoy once you're free. You don't have to worry about any of this any more.

If you're reading this worrying you might have 'done all the damage already', please don't. There is not an illness or disease known to man where quitting nicotine doesn't dramatically improve the prognosis many, many times over, to quite an extraordinary extent.

The nicotine trap is unrelenting: the more you consume, the more you want to consume; the less you consume, the more you want to consume. It's like tying someone up, so that the slightest movement tightens the rope around their neck.

OCCASIONAL VAPERS

But what about those casual vapers who seem so cool and relaxed that it's impossible to believe they're suffering? I'm talking about the ones who can go for days without vaping and just do it every now and then. In the eyes of other vapers, these lucky people really have got their vaping under control. They seem to have been spared the misery of addiction. The truth is very different and you can unveil it by asking them one simple question:

WHAT'S THE POINT?

If they think they're getting some genuine pleasure or crutch from occasional vaping, why wait so long in between? If they don't get any genuine pleasure or crutch, why vape at all?

If you're a heavy vaper who envies occasional vapers, have you ever tried cutting down?

If so, what was it like? Every time I ask a heavy vaper the same question they reply that it was hell, or words to that effect.

Vapers who go for weeks without doing it don't even suffer the illusion of getting pleasure or a crutch from vaping, they just go through the motions to be part of the company. All vapers started off like that, convinced that they would never get hooked. They're like a fly hovering around the lip of the pitcher plant and they often turn into full-on vapers.

If you think it sounds appealing to only want to vape once every now and then, wouldn't it be even better never to want to do it at all? All vapers who restrict their intake are creating a number of serious problems for themselves:

- They keep themselves physically addicted to nicotine. This keeps their brain craving vape.

- They wish their lives away waiting for the next fix.

- Instead of vaping whenever they feel like it and partially relieving their craving most of the time, they force themselves to suffer constant mental aggravation and conflict.

• They reinforce the illusion that vaping is enjoyable.

Cutting down increases the illusion of pleasure because the longer you crave nicotine, the more marvellous it feels when you relieve the craving. 'What's so bad about that?' you might ask. Because it's not genuine pleasure, it's relief from discomfort, like wearing tight shoes for the pleasure of taking them off. The only way to increase the illusion of pleasure is to increase the discomfort.

No vaper enjoys that discomfort – and casual vapers have to endure it longer than other vapers. Casual vaping is rarely sustainable. The addiction makes you want to scratch the itch, not suffer it, and the tendency is to vape more and more.

Casual vaping is a terrible form of slavery. You're constantly using willpower to restrict the amount you vape and perpetually thinking about whether or not you will allow yourself to do it. Get it clear in your mind:

YOU DON'T CONTROL YOUR VAPING; IT CONTROLS YOU!

Most vapers know from experience that cutting down doesn't help you quit. On the contrary, it usually leaves you feeling more addicted. It's much easier to escape the trap by stopping outright. There's no need for half measures. Why would you want to vape for the rest of your life, when you can be free of the whole filthy nightmare?

STOPPERS AND STARTERS

Casual vapers and occasional vapers have the worst of both worlds: they can neither vape when they want to nor do they have the wonderful joy of being free. The same is true of stop-start vapers.

This type of vaper is also envied by heavier vapers, because they appear to have control over their vaping, in the same way that occasional vapers seem to. Not wanting to appear stupid, they encourage the misconception – but, of course, it's a lie.

Think about it: if these vapers truly enjoy doing it, why do they keep stopping? And if they don't enjoy being vapers, why do they keep starting again? The answer is very obvious: they don't enjoy being vapers and they don't enjoy being non-vapers either. How tragic! Trapped in a kind of purgatory, repeatedly going through the trauma of quitting and the misery and self-loathing of starting again.

To be a happy non-vaper for the rest of your life, you need to achieve the right frame of mind. If you believe you're making a sacrifice, you will always feel deprived. If you regard just one vape as a pleasure or crutch, you'll remain vulnerable for the rest of your life.

Easyway makes it easy to quit completely and permanently by helping you to remove any desire to vape. That doesn't mean you can vape occasionally and use the method to get free again. If you feel the desire for 'just the one' vape, then the Big Monster is still alive, you haven't removed the brainwashing and you still believe the myth. Even a casual 'just one' will raise the Big Monster from his grave.

Our mission is to remove your desire to take even a single puff of a vape, because if you want one you will want a million. Even if you resist the temptation to have that single puff but merely desire it, you will not be a happy 'non-vaper'. You will be a miserable 'ex-vaper'. Eventually, when your willpower runs out, you will cease to be a miserable ex-vaper and will become an even more miserable vaper.

And the most miserable vaper of all is...

THE SECRET VAPER

Secret vapers can't even pretend that they enjoy it. They steal furtive drags when they think nobody is looking. They're not kidding anyone except themselves.

Does that ring a bell? You tell your loved ones you're going to quit but don't and then start lying to cover it up. Breaking the promise is bad enough, but to compound that by lying is the ultimate humiliation.

If you vape openly you can at least claim that you do it because you choose to. As a secret vaper you have to admit to yourself that you're just a slave to nicotine. Secret vapers go through life despising themselves. People with great integrity find themselves lying to conceal their shame. They even start believing their own lies.

This is what the addiction does to you. When you've tried as hard as you can to cut down or quit and still you find yourself helplessly drawn back to it, the confusion, despair and shame make a liar of you. But although you lie to your loved ones and to yourself, underneath you remain acutely aware of the painful truth: you're a slave to nicotine, a miserable, pathetic drug addict.

ALL VAPERS ARE THE SAME

It doesn't matter what type of vaper you think you are, all vapers, all nicotine addicts, have something fundamental in common:

THEY ALL WISH THEY HAD NEVER STARTED

You have no reason to envy any of them. They are all victims of the trap from which you are trying to escape. And you're doing well. You are nearly ready to complete your escape and eventually to feel the moment of revelation.

Every type of nicotine addict would love to wake up in the morning in the position you'll be in soon:

FREE

Chapter 15

VAPING QUESTIONS

IN THIS CHAPTER

•THE TRUTH ABOUT VAPING •THE MOMENT OF REVELATION
•WILL THE GOOD TIMES STILL ROLL? •WILL THE HARD TIMES HURT MORE?
•NICOTINE DOESN'T FILL A VOID – IT CREATES ONE •ARE YOU READY?

Unravelling the brainwashing is not hard but it does require commitment and an open mind. You need to digest what you've learned and change your mindset from the belief that vaping or any other nicotine product provides some sort of pleasure or benefit to the total understanding that it does nothing for you at all. As you look forward to testing your newfound knowledge, some questions will arise. I'm happy to answer those now.

THE TRUTH ABOUT VAPING

Congratulations on getting to this point. Most nicotine addicts go through their lives oblivious to the understanding that you have gained while reading this book. You are in a very powerful position. Not only do you hold the keys to your prison, you now have the knowledge to use them.

You may already feel absolutely clear in your mind that you no longer have any desire to vape or take nicotine in any form and that you feel you're ready to quit. If so, resist the temptation to skip to the final vape. You might miss something vital. If you still harbour some, or even a lot of, uncertainty about your ability to quit, don't worry, that's perfectly natural. Take the time and care to finish the book. Regardless of whether you can believe it or not at this stage, you'll be a happy non-vaper in no time at all.

As we prepare for your last moments as a nicotine addict, let's recap everything you've learned.

THERE IS NO PLEASURE IN VAPING

There is only the illusion of pleasure. Any perceived enjoyment is merely temporary and partial relief from the empty, insecure feeling of nicotine withdrawing from your body.

That triggers a thought process in your mind which makes you feel more and more deprived and makes the illusory relief appear even greater.

Vaping to achieve that feeling is like wearing tight shoes just to get the relief of taking them off. It's like being grateful to the thief for returning £10 of the £100 he secretly stole from you. Would you be grateful in those circumstances once you discovered what he'd done?

YOU DON'T NEED WILLPOWER TO QUIT

You only need willpower when you have a conflict of wills. Remove the desire to vape and you lose any sense that you're depriving yourself when you quit. Believe that you're making a sacrifice and you will always be vulnerable to starting again.

THERE IS NO SUCH THING AS AN ADDICTIVE PERSONALITY

If you think you have addictive traits, it's because you became hooked on an addictive drug, not the other way around. Even if you're convinced that you have an addictive personality or genes, the great news is that you'll still find it easy to get free. This addiction is easy to break when you know how... regardless of genes and personality.

NICOTINE DOES NOT HELP YOU CONCENTRATE

It actually makes it harder. Nicotine addiction is a constant distraction. The Little Monster starts crying for its next fix as soon as you start withdrawing from the previous dose, and it becomes impossible to concentrate on anything else until you satisfy the craving.

NICOTINE DOES NOT EASE STRESS

Nicotine addiction is a major cause of stress. The constant desire to vape, no matter how slight, means you are never fully relaxed. Any sense of relaxation you get when vaping is just the partial relief of the discomfort of withdrawing from the previous shot of the drug and the ending of the mental aggravation the Big Monster causes. It is temporary, and as you put your vaping device down the discomfort creeps back in. Quit vaping, get free of the Little Monster and the Big Monster and your overall stress levels will fall considerably.

ALL NICOTINE ADDICTS LIE

Pay no attention to what nicotine addicts say, whether it's about the supposed benefits of vaping or nicotine in any form or the terrible trauma of quitting. Nicotine addicts lie to cover up their sense of shame and helplessness. You know the truth. See through the illusions and fix your mind on the true picture.

VAPING IS NOT FREEDOM

Anyone who argues that the choice to vape is down to the rights of the individual fails to understand addiction. You don't vape out of choice; you vape to feed your addiction. Vaping controls the addict, not the other way round. It's not freedom; it's slavery.

THE GLAMOUR OF SCREEN STARS ISN'T REAL

The powerful influence of famous role models attracts millions of people to smoking and vaping. When you see a big celebrity photographed vaping, it's easy to forget that they too are suffering with the nervousness, irritability, stress, ill health and slavery of nicotine addiction. They make vaping appear cool – it's not the other way around.

SUBSTITUTES DON'T WORK

Replacing vaping with another source of nicotine, or vice versa, is guaranteed to keep you addicted. Using a substitute to gradually cut down on your nicotine intake actually makes quitting harder. As you restrict your intake, so the sense of deprivation increases and the drug seems more precious. The easy way to quit is to unravel the myth that nicotine gives you some sort of pleasure or crutch, remove any desire to vape or take it in any other form and stop completely.

NEITHER SMOKING NOR VAPING KEEPS YOU THIN

Most heavy smokers and vapers are overweight. They are constantly suffering the empty feeling of withdrawal from nicotine, which feels just like hunger. When they're not smoking or vaping, they're eating. Neither satisfies the craving for the other. When you quit with Easyway, you recognise that the empty, insecure feeling of withdrawal is not painful, it's the barely perceptible death throes of the Little Monster, and you know that eating won't make it go away. After a few days the Little Monster dies and you're free from the feeling for good.

ALL VAPERS ARE THE SAME

There is no reason to envy other vapers for the amount they do or don't vape. All vapers are in the same trap, controlled by the drug and constantly fighting the urge to do it more. If you think you can get away with vaping occasionally, ask yourself this: 'Why would I want to?' If you answer, 'Because it will give me pleasure or a crutch', then you haven't seen through the myth. Don't panic… the rest of the book is designed to ensure that you do.

NICOTINE DOES ABSOLUTELY NOTHING WHATSOEVER FOR YOU

You need to be absolutely clear on this. Before you have your final shot of nicotine, you have to make sure the Big Monster that interprets the cries of the Little Monster as 'I want a vape' is dead. Otherwise, you will be forever drawing on your willpower to fight the temptation to do it. With Easyway, you remove the temptation altogether. When you finish your final vape, you will have no remaining desire to do it ever again.

HOW WILL I KNOW WHEN I'M A HAPPY NON-NICOTINE ADDICT?

This is the most common question vapers ask when they're attempting to quit. How will I know when I've succeeded? It's natural to ask this question because most vapers will have tried to quit before, using willpower, and will know the feeling of uncertainty that dogs you with that method.

People make their own assumptions. A particular vaper might say: 'I'll know I'm a happy non-vaper when...'

- '... I can go out drinking with my friends or enjoy a meal without wanting to vape.'
- '... I've managed to go a whole day without vaping.'
- '... I feel like a non-vaper.'

In each case, the vaper assumes that they will have to get through an initial period of feeling deprived – and they have no idea how long that may last.

With the willpower method, you never know when you've succeeded in quitting because you are constantly waiting for something to happen – the moment when you give in and vape. All you can do is hope it won't happen. Sadly, in the vast majority of cases, it happens all too soon.

With Easyway, the uncertainty is removed. You don't have to wait for anything. You become a happy non-vaper the moment you finish your final vape. Killing the Big Monster means achieving absolute certainty that you will never desire another vape in your life. This is how a non-vaper feels. They are aware of vapes – they may even believe part of the myth – but they have absolutely no desire whatsoever to vape.

The only reason anyone continues to vape is to relieve the withdrawal pangs created by the previous shot of the drug.

Once you have this clearly in your mind, it's easy to unravel the rest of the brainwashing and kill the Big Monster. With Easyway, you kill the Big Monster before having your final vape. With the willpower method, you kill the Little Monster and hope the Big Monster will leave you alone. But as long as the Big Monster remains alive and you believe that there is some pleasure or crutch to be derived from nicotine, you will never be free.

LET ME EXPLAIN WHY IT DOESN'T MATTER IF YOU HAVE A WILLPOWER ISSUE

THE OINTMENT ANALOGY

Imagine you have a cold sore on your face. I tell you that I have this marvellous ointment.

I say to you: 'Try this stuff, it's brilliant.' You put the ointment on and the cold sore disappears immediately.

A week later, the cold sore reappears. You come back to me and say: 'Can I have some more of that ointment?' Again, you apply the ointment and, miraculously, the sore disappears. I say to you: 'Keep the tube, you might need it again.'

The process continues, but every time it comes back the cold sore gets bigger and more painful, and the interval gets shorter and shorter.

Eventually, the sore is the size of your head and is returning every half hour. Now you know the ointment will give temporary relief, but you are now terribly worried.

What is this awful disease? Will it eventually spread all over my body? Will the ointment cease to give even temporary relief? You go to your doctor, but he can't cure it. You try other remedies, but nothing will help, just this marvellous ointment.

You would feel completely dependent on that ointment. You would never go out without making sure that you had a tube. Now, in addition to worrying about your health, I am charging you £100 for each tube and you are having difficulty in finding the money.

You then read an article in your newspaper and discover this is not only happening to you. Thousands of other people are using this ointment and it has been proved that, far from curing the cold sore, it is the ointment that is causing it to grow. All the ointment does is take the initial sore beneath the skin and then the sore feeds on the ointment. All you have to do to get rid of the cold sore is to stop using the ointment and the sore will disappear of its own accord.

Would you use that ointment again?
Of course you wouldn't!
Would it take willpower not to use it again?
No!
Would you be miserable?
Again no!

If you have any doubts about that at all, try to imagine the position I have described. You were going to die and you had no solution. Now you have found the solution, you are not going to die. You would not be miserable – you would be elated. If you did not believe that the ointment was causing the sore, there might be a few days of apprehension during which you would have to wait for the evidence to confirm the truth. But as you saw the cold sore gradually disappearing, you would be overjoyed to realise that you had found the answer to the problem.

This was the so-called magic that happened to me all those years ago, when I got free. Let me make it quite clear. In the analogy to vaping, the cold sore is not cancer, or lung damage, or the stigma, or the tens of thousands of pounds we waste, or the lifetime of lethargy, or the slavery or the deprivation. These are all in addition to the cold sore. The cold sore is this panic feeling of: 'I want a vape.' Non-vapers do not suffer that panic feeling and this is what blocks our minds from all the other horrors. Nicotine does not relieve that panic feeling. The first shot of the drug starts it, and all the others do is to make sure that you suffer it again and again and again.

When I got free I could see that the panic feeling of wanting nicotine was not a weakness in me, and that it was caused by the previous dose of the drug. The one thing that would stop it going away was the next dose of the drug.

THE MOMENT OF REVELATION

So far I've dedicated much of our time to helping you rewire your brain, enabling you to change your mindset from one of wanting to vape to one of moving towards having no desire to vape whatsoever. The same applies to whichever form of nicotine addiction you suffer.

Don't worry if you don't think you've moved towards that mindset yet – all will become clear.

Achieving this change of mindset is a simple process of unravelling the brainwashing step by step, examining the myths that surround nicotine addiction and dismantling them one by one.

If you think there are still some illusions that you haven't quite seen through, don't worry. By the end of the book you will be in a position to have your final dose of nicotine and rather than having a feeling of foreboding you'll be delighted to be free. Give yourself time while we continue to

REWIRE YOUR BRAIN

I fully expect the remainder of the book to handle every single query or concern that you might have remaining.

While killing the Big Monster is a simple process, there is nothing unusual or stupid about having to go over certain points more than once. It's much better that you achieve complete certainty over each point than rush to the end. There is also nothing unusual or stupid about believing that quitting nicotine is one of the hardest things to do. We are all brainwashed into believing that, and the efforts of other vapers to quit through willpower appear to confirm it. You may even have seemed to prove it to yourself with your own previous efforts.

And so you may have reached this point fully understanding everything you've heard, yet still feeling apprehensive about your own ability to quit. Somewhere in your mind you suspect that it can't be this easy – there must be a major hurdle waiting to trip you up.

THE ONLY THING THAT CAN STOP YOU NOW IS YOUR OWN DISBELIEF

Seeing through illusions means believing the evidence of your own eyes. Set aside everything you have ever been told about vaping or any form of nicotine and look at it logically. If you have understood everything about nicotine addiction, about the trap and the myths that keep addicts believing they're getting some pleasure or crutch from the drug, then all you have to do now is allow yourself to believe.

THERE IS NO CATCH

It really is that simple. Once you understand beyond all doubt that vaping, far from relieving the empty feeling, causes it, you have already removed the cause of panic at the thought of quitting.

You are on the brink of achieving something remarkable. It could be the most life-changing thing you've ever done. You now know that everything you've ever been led to believe about the perceived benefits of nicotine, or the difficulty involved in quitting, was a lie. The moment when all this knowledge falls into place and all doubt is removed is the moment when the Big Monster dies. We call it 'the moment of revelation'. For some people it is a huge thrill, like a blinding flash of light, a sudden realisation of the truth and the opening of a prison door. For others, it is little more than the completion of a circle, a logical conclusion that enables them to calmly finish their final vape and get on with life as a happy non-nicotine addict. For some, it doesn't happen until a few days or even weeks after they've quit. It suddenly dawns on them, maybe after an event or incident that might have caused them to vape in the past. 'WOW! I'm free! I didn't even think about vaping!' In either case, don't wait for it to happen while you're reading this book or even afterwards; one thing I can assure you of is that *you* will have that moment. Enjoy it.

WILL THE GOOD TIMES STILL ROLL?

As a vaper, you believed that vaping provided you with a pleasure and a crutch. No doubt you had your 'special' vapes, such as the first one you had after a meal. These are the occasions vapers fear they'll miss the most and they formulate the notion that the good times will cease to roll if they're not able to cap them with a vape.

The notion of 'special' vapes is a vaper's fantasy.

One vaper who came to our seminar in New York explained that the one thing holding him back was the thought that he would never be able to sit outside a café in Paris, watching the crowds go by, sipping a glass of wine and vaping. On further investigation it transpired that the man had never even been to Paris, let alone been in that situation. It was all a fantasy, probably something he'd seen in a film. Yet he couldn't bear the thought of never doing it. He was moping for a myth.

If you're fortunate enough to find yourself in Paris on a sunny day, take a seat outside a café, order a drink, watch the crowds go by and see how it feels. You'll find it has all the charm and appeal anyone could imagine and is all the better for not having to pollute the moment with vape.

Those so-called 'special' vapes only seem special because they come after a prolonged period of abstinence – sleep, eating, a game of sport, etc. Think back over your time as a vaper and try to remember a single moment that made you think: 'I'm so glad to be a vaper.' I'm sure you'll remember many that stirred the opposite feeling, vaping moments that made you feel utterly miserable because you'd vaped too much or were simply embarrassed by the need to vape.

You will no doubt remember occasions, too, when you felt utterly miserable because you weren't allowed to vape, and how relieved you were when you finally got to do so, but that's different. If you're honest, you'll find that the only occasions when you're truly aware of your vaping are when you want to do it but can't, or when you're vaping but wish you didn't have to. If you continue believing that you can't enjoy certain situations without vaping, then you won't.

Part of the process of changing your mindset is recognising that nicotine does not enhance good times, it taints them. You need to turn your belief around so that this is clear. Analyse the situations I've described to understand why the vaping or JUUL or IQOS or dip or snus appears to enhance them but actually does the opposite.

As a happy non-nicotine addict, you will enjoy the good times in life more. You will feel more relaxed without nicotine withdrawal, you won't have the anxiety of making sure you're stocked up with vape, you won't have to worry about spoiling the enjoyment of other people by blowing vapour all over them... plus, you'll have the immense satisfaction of knowing that you are free from the awful slavery of the nicotine addict.

WILL THE HARD TIMES HURT MORE?

Let's be honest about this, no one goes through life without some hardship and pain. It is perfectly normal. Our aim is not to protect you from ever suffering again; that would be utterly unrealistic. But by becoming a non-nicotine addict, you will be more resilient when fate turns against you.

Nicotine addicts believe that the drug provides a crutch – something they can lean on to help them through life's hardships. A typical scenario is a car breakdown. It's late at night, pouring with rain, you're on the most dangerous part of the road, your phone has no signal and all the other drivers on the road are hurrying past at high speed, rather than stopping to see if they can help. Some of them are even tooting at you, as if you've chosen to park your car there for the fun of it.

It's a miserable, forlorn situation and a vaper would reach for a vape, thinking it would give them some respite from the stress and misery. The challenge arises the next time you're in this situation, after having become a non-vaper. Miserable and angry, you think to yourself: 'At times like this I would have had a vape.' It's a crucial moment and you must be prepared for it.

Look back at the last time you faced such a crisis and vaped. Did vaping solve your problem? Did you have a sudden change of mood and stand there in the rain happily thinking, 'Never mind the car or the fact that I'm wet and miserable, I've got this marvellous vape!'? Or were you still utterly miserable? If you think at that time you were consoled by the vape, that's the thief giving you £10 of the £100 he stole. A non-vaper in that situation can focus on the situation and doesn't have to worry about running out of vape or whether they can vape or not.

When people who have quit with the willpower method find themselves in these situations, they start to mope for nicotine. They don't realise that nicotine, far from helping the situation, actually makes it worse by adding extra layers of stress to an already stressful situation.

As part of your change of mindset, make sure you accept that there will be ups and downs in life, just as there are for other non-nicotine addicts, and that if you think nicotine will help at such times you will be moping for an illusion, grasping for something that does not exist and creating a void. Be absolutely clear – removing nicotine from your life does not leave a void.

NICOTINE DOESN'T FILL A VOID – IT CREATES ONE

Ex-nicotine addicts who don't understand this suffer the misery of turning good days into bad days and making bad days worse. With Easyway, you turn your mindset around so you can do the opposite. You won't miss vaping or any form of nicotine and you will enjoy life more. You will be better equipped to deal with the natural stresses and anxieties that life throws up. And no matter how bad life gets, you will always be able to pick yourself up with the thought

YIPPEE! I'M FREE!

ARE YOU READY?

It's not just crisis situations that can trigger the thought of vaping. Happy occasions like birthdays, Christmas, weddings and holidays are also likely to stir memories of your vaping days. It's nothing to worry about. All you have to do is be prepared for them.

Ex-nicotine addicts who quit with the willpower method are easily caught off guard. The temptation to vape in social situations like weddings can be overwhelming if you still believe that you will be missing out if you don't vape. Take some time to think about the occasions and moments in life that might be a trigger for you and then prepare your response in advance.

In any situation when your thoughts might turn to vaping, instead of thinking,

'I USED TO HAVE A VAPE IN THIS SITUATION,'

think,

'ISN'T IT MARVELLOUS! I NO LONGER HAVE TO VAPE. I'M FREE!'

That way you will turn any association between the occasion and vaping to your advantage, reinforcing the truth that nicotine does absolutely nothing for you and that you have no need or desire to vape.

We have devoted this book to replacing illusions with truths. All you need to do now is convince yourself that you don't just understand those truths but that you believe them wholeheartedly. Remember, once you see through an illusion you cannot be fooled by it again.

There is nothing waiting to trip you up. Allow yourself to feel an incredible sense of excitement. You are on the brink of a fantastic achievement. Like a prisoner who knows that release awaits them, think about all the wonderful benefits that freedom will bring: better health, more money, greater self-esteem, less stress, better concentration, no fear, no guilt, no slavery. Or, to put it another way,

TOTAL HAPPINESS

Recap everything that you've learned so far. Go over all the myths and make sure you are completely clear, seeing things as they really are, not through the distorted lens of addiction and brainwashing.

You're approaching a huge moment in your life – the moment you have your final dose of nicotine and become a happy non-addict for life. Congratulate yourself on reaching this point. Millions of nicotine addicts would love to be in the position you're in now, holding the key to your own prison cell. Ask yourself a couple of last questions:

DO I WANT TO USE THE KEY?

OR

DO I WANT TO REMAIN A SLAVE FOR THE REST OF MY LIFE?

There can be only one answer, the one all nicotine addicts would give if they possessed the knowledge that you now have.

PREPARE YOURSELF FOR FREEDOM

Chapter 16

THE BIGGEST MOMENT OF YOUR LIFE

IN THIS CHAPTER

NICOTINE DOES NOTHING FOR YOU *REAL VS IMAGINARY FEARS*
NO NEED FOR A SAFETY NET *MAKE YOUR CHOICE*
REWIRE YOUR BRAIN *FREE FROM THE NIGHTMARE*

You are approaching the biggest moment of your life. I do not exaggerate! Perhaps you feel you've had more important days: the day you were born perhaps; the day you fell in love; got married; had your children. These are all momentous, happy days that change your life – but the approaching moment will save your life.

Let me remind you again of my fourth instruction:

THINK POSITIVELY

In other words:

BEGIN, NOT WITH A FEELING OF DOOM AND GLOOM, BUT INSTEAD WITH A FEELING OF ELATION AND EXCITEMENT.

Bear in mind, I'm not saying: 'Kid yourself into thinking that everything is going to be OK and the chances of everything being OK will be greatly improved (even though it's going to be tough as hell).' I'm saying everything is going to be OK.

More than OK in fact. All you need to do is avoid bracing yourself in anticipation of having problems. If you expect problems, every slight bump in the road feels like a catastrophe and causes panic. You're going to find it ridiculously easy to quit nicotine – so just assume that's the way it's going to be and look forward to freedom.

You have nothing to lose from that approach and everything to gain.

If I was asking you to step off a tall building and trust that I can make you fly – I'd fully understand your very sensible reluctance to trust me. You'd be staking your life in your trust for me. But I'm not asking you to do anything dangerous or foolhardy or reckless and the risks of trusting me are minimal. You're a nicotine addict. What's the very worst thing that could happen as a result of you assuming that everything is going to be fine after you quit? Nothing! You'll either find it easy to quit or you won't. If you quit and it's easy – great. If you fail and carry on vaping, JUULing, chewing, or snusing, you'll be no worse off than you are now.

NOTHING BAD IS GOING TO HAPPEN AFTER YOU QUIT. QUITE THE CONTRARY.

Shortly you will take your final dose of nicotine, and you will do so with the absolute certainty you will never want more. Just think what that means – you will never again suffer the slavery and degradation of being a nicotine addict. Everybody has different things that they look forward to most when they are on the brink of becoming free from nicotine addiction. Some look forward to feeling healthier and being free from any side effects they've noticed – the headaches and the nervous fidgets. Some look forward to having more money to spend on genuine pleasures.

Some can't wait to tell their family and friends, bringing an end to all the guilt and regaining their self-respect. Some just want to take back control of their lives.

Being free from nicotine addiction provides so many bonuses that are exciting and wonderful and joyous, but the most important one of all is this:

FREEDOM FROM THE SLAVERY

All nicotine addicts know the arguments for not using nicotine and can't understand why they find it so hard to quit. They don't understand the nature of the trap they're in and the fact that they're addicted to nicotine. And so they feel enslaved by some unknown force that compels them to keep taking it against their better judgement.

But you *do* understand the trap and you know that the only reason you have continued to vape is because of nicotine addiction. Now you have the key to unlock your chains and be free. Remember, you're doing this for yourself. It is you who is being freed from slavery and all you need to think about is your own journey. Everything else will fall into place.

Shortly I will lead you to the thrilling moment when you have your final dose of nicotine – or if you quit before finishing this book, you can confirm that you have already had your final dose.

Then you'll walk free from the nicotine trap for good. Allow yourself to feel very excited. Remind yourself of everything you stand to gain and of everything you now know about the myths and illusions and the brainwashing that creates them.

Focus on those two monsters inside you and prepare to unleash your vengeance on them for all the misery they've caused you.

ARE YOU READY?

LET'S GO!

THERE IS NOTHING TO FEAR

AS YOU APPROACH THE MOMENT WHEN YOU HAVE YOUR FINAL VAPE – YOUR FINAL DOSE OF NICOTINE – IT'S NATURAL TO FEEL BUTTERFLIES IN YOUR STOMACH AND MISTAKE THIS FOR THE FEAR OF SUCCESS. REMEMBER, FEAR PLAYS A VERY VALUABLE ROLE IN YOUR SURVIVAL TOOLKIT, BUT THE FEAR OF BEING A NON-NICOTINE ADDICT IS COMPLETELY IRRATIONAL.

NICOTINE DOES NOTHING FOR YOU

When you first started this book you were under the impression that you derived some pleasure or benefit from nicotine and you were looking for help in overcoming your need for that pleasure or crutch. As you've worked through the book, you have turned your understanding of nicotine addiction on its head, so you should now be very clear on a number of facts that are the complete opposite of what vapers – and in fact all nicotine addicts – believe, such as:

**VAPING OR ANY OTHER FORM OF NICOTINE CONSUMPTION
DOESN'T RELIEVE YOUR CRAVING; IT CAUSES IT.**

NICOTINE DOESN'T EASE STRESS; IT IS A MAJOR CAUSE OF STRESS.

YOU DON'T CONTROL NICOTINE; IT CONTROLS YOU.

At our Easyway seminars, we are often asked: 'If vaping does nothing
for you whatsoever, why tell us to keep doing it until the final dose?'

It is a sensible question. Again, you need to turn it on its head. It is
important for you to keep vaping as you progress through the book,
not because of what vaping does for you but for what happens to you
when you don't do it.

The Big Monster tells you 'I want to vape' as the nicotine from the
previous dose withdraws from your body. If you're not allowed to
vape, you become fidgety and distracted. This inability to concentrate
is caused by nicotine, so we need to make sure that you aren't
distracted from the task in hand because of that. Once you've had
your final dose of nicotine, your concentration will no longer be
disturbed by the addiction, but until that time it's important that you
continue to consume nicotine as you normally would.

REAL VS IMAGINARY FEARS

Nicotine addicts don't need to be told that it's a mug's game. That's
an old English expression for 'you're the mark in the scam'. They are
perfectly capable of weighing up the advantages and disadvantages
and concluding that they would be much better off not being addicted,
yet they also know that the force which compels them to carry on is

very real. Moreover, they know what it feels like when they don't respond to that force.

No one wants to spend the rest of their life feeling the way a nicotine addict feels when they can't have their drug, and this is why they fear the thought of becoming free. What they don't realise is that nicotine causes that feeling and the only way to be completely rid of it is to stop taking the drug.

Fear is the force that keeps you in the trap. It feeds on all the brainwashing and myths that you've been bombarded with from an early age. It's important to recognise that this fear is caused by the addiction to nicotine, as distinct from the genuine, instinctive fears that form a vital part of your survival toolkit.

The instinctive fears that protect us from fire, falling, drowning, etc., are all perfectly logical. The fear of not being able to vape is completely illogical. It is a fear based on your imagination, which is clouded by illusions. People who don't vape don't suffer from it at all.

THE FEAR OF BEING FREE OF NICOTINE WAS CREATED WHEN YOU STARTED VAPING

For addicts still caught in the nicotine trap, however, this fear is very real. The willpower method advises them to fight through the fear, when it's obvious that what they really need is to have their eyes opened to the fact that the fear is not founded in reality. Easyway removes the fear by showing you that there is nothing to fear and there is no sacrifice, no deprivation, no pain and no discomfort whatsoever. Nicotine does absolutely nothing for you at all and when you stop, all the things you think you're going to miss evaporate. But you don't have to wait until you are a non-nicotine addict to make the fear disappear. You can easily remove it by approaching the subject with an open mind and trying to be relaxed, logical and rational. Then you will be able to see the truth through the illusions and you will have no reason to fear life without nicotine.

NO NEED FOR A SAFETY NET

Once they realise that it's just fear that prevents them from stopping, some vapers try to set their fear aside by telling themselves that they can always start vaping again if they're finding it hard – quitting doesn't have to be final. This is a big mistake. If you start off with that attitude, you're very likely to be dragged back into the trap.

High-wire artists who don't use a safety net may be adding an extra element of drama to their act, but there is more to it than that. They will use a safety net during practice, because they are not yet certain that they have perfected their routine. However, by the time of the performance they are so certain of their act and their ability to carry it off that the presence of a safety net would actually be a hindrance – sowing a seed of doubt in their mind, which can throw them off balance.

The same applies with your own great act – escape from the nicotine trap. In order to walk free easily, painlessly and permanently, you must have complete certainty about what you're doing. Telling yourself you can always take up vaping again if you're struggling is like quitting with a safety net.

The whole point of a safety net is that it should go unused. The great thing about becoming free is that there's no danger. You're not going to fall and hurt yourself; nothing bad is going to happen. You simply don't need a safety net any more than you would need a handrail to walk across an empty room. The certainty you need is happening in your mind. Perhaps you think nothing in life is ever certain. After all, the chances of being hit by a meteorite are infinitesimally small, yet there remains a possibility that it could happen. OK, that's true. But here's the difference. If a meteorite is going to hit you, there is absolutely nothing you can do about it. It's not your decision, whereas putting nicotine into your body is entirely your decision. As long as you don't make that decision, you can be absolutely certain that it won't happen.

Q: WHY DOES ANYONE EVER LET NICOTINE INTO THEIR BODY? A: BECAUSE THEY WANT TO

Wait a minute! Earlier I restated the fact that you don't control nicotine, nicotine controls you. Doesn't this go against the answer just provided? That you only let nicotine into your body because you want to?

This brings us to the key to quitting with Easyway. As a vaper, JUULer, IQOSer, snuser, dipper or gum or tobacco chewer, you choose when you take every single dose of nicotine. Nobody else forces you to do it. Yet it's what controls the choices you make that makes the difference. It's nicotine addiction that controls your choice.

Free from addiction, it's easy to make the choice not to do it. It's in your hands. When you finish your final dose of nicotine, you can be absolutely certain that you will never let it into your body again. All you have to do is make sure you are never again sidetracked by the thought 'I want a vape'. You can achieve this by making sure you have three vital facts ingrained in your mind:

1. Vaping, or any nicotine product, does absolutely nothing for you whatsoever. You must understand why this is. That way you will have no feeling of deprivation.

2. You don't need to go through any transitional period (often referred to incorrectly as the 'withdrawal period') before the craving goes completely. Craving is mental, not physical, and yours will be gone by the time you've finished this book. What's more, the physical withdrawal is so slight it's hardly perceptible.

3. There is no such thing as 'one vape' or 'one dose of nicotine'. Never think in terms of one dose; think of a hundred thousand doses, a lifetime's chain of control, mood swings, slavery and misery.

MAKE YOUR CHOICE

A lot of nicotine addicts find it hard to believe that they have a choice about whether to crave the drug or not. They are trapped by the misconception that you either crave something or you don't, and there's nothing you can do about it. Fortunately, they're wrong. Your body will continue to experience nicotine withdrawal for a few days after quitting as the Little Monster goes through its death throes, but that doesn't mean you have to be miserable or that you have to crave nicotine.

How you respond to the Little Monster dying is completely up to you. The physical feeling is very slight, the mildest feeling you can imagine, no more alarming than, out of the corner of your eye, noticing a bit of fluff on your shoulder. At first it might surprise you, but after a moment you'd simply respond by gently brushing the fluff away. You wouldn't panic nor would you worry about the next piece of fluff that might land on your shoulder.

It's the Big Monster in your mind that reacts to the mild feeling by creating a mental process which, in turn, causes more troubling physical feelings. The great news is that once you've changed your mental reaction to the mild physical feelings, the thought processes become enjoyable rather than bothersome.

The discomfort you've experienced in the past has been based on the following thought process triggered by the mild withdrawal feeling:

'I WANT A VAPE!'
'I CAN'T HAVE ONE!'
'AGHHH!'

If there is no pleasure, benefit or crutch obtained from nicotine, then you won't want any nicotine. True? Of course it is.

If you don't *want* nicotine, then you won't feel that you *can't* have it, and then you won't have that 'AGHHH!' feeling. True? Of course it is.

I don't feel that I *'can't have'* porridge for breakfast. I'm not interested in porridge. I can guarantee that at no point in my life will the thought of me not having porridge make me feel 'AGHHH'.

Now whether you love porridge or loathe it, don't let that stand in the way of understanding where I'm coming from. If you understand that something has absolutely nothing to offer you, you will need to make no effort whatsoever to abstain from it.

If you understand that, just on principle, then you're on the verge of becoming a happy non-nicotine addict.

If after you quit you ever feel that you're having that 'I want a vape' thought, please don't worry. After months or years of doing it, it wouldn't be surprising. Remember, it's just like spotting a bit of fluff out of the corner of your eye on your shoulder. Just brush it off and don't let it send you into a panic. All it means is that you momentarily forgot that you quit; it doesn't mean you want to vape. No more than nearly taking a wrong turn on your way home from work towards your old apartment means that you want to move out of the amazing apartment you moved into recently. It just takes some time for our brains to get used to our new situation. I'll come back to this issue later on and in doing so I'll explain why *thinking about* nicotine, specifically thinking '*I want a vape*', or any other form of nicotine, may have made it so hard, or even impossible, for you to quit in the past. And in turn I'll explain why this time, by rewiring your brain, you're all set to find it easy .

The willpower method encourages nicotine addicts to fixate on the craving by making it the focus of their resistance. They have to use their willpower to try to avoid thinking about vaping and resist reaching for nicotine. If you've ever made a conscious effort to NOT think about something, you'll know what a futile exercise this is. Let's try it now.

If I say, 'Whatever you do now don't think about a pink elephant!', what is the first thing you do? Exactly, no doubt you've got a picture of a pink elephant in your mind.

With Easyway, you can choose to brush off the Little Monster completely. It's really not hard – the feeling is so slight. Or you can choose to rejoice in the feeling – after all, it signals the death of a mortal enemy. This is a very important point. Many vapers are convinced that nicotine is their friend, their crutch, their source of confidence and courage, even part of their identity. They fear that quitting will hit them like losing a close friend and maybe even a part of themselves. That's why these vapers become whining ex-vapers. But their behaviour is very different to genuine grief.

When you lose a close friend, you mourn, you suffer shock and there's a huge sense of loss at the initial tragedy. But, to an extent, you recover from this shock and get on with life. The loss leaves a void in your life that can never be filled, you rightly keep your special memories of your friend alive and look back fondly, but you have no choice other than to accept the situation and eventually you do.

But you're not losing a friend. As a friend it would be most peculiar; it stinks, controls your every move, steals your money, won't leave you alone and is trying to kill you. That's not a friend. It's an enemy!

When you rid yourself of a mortal enemy, there is no mourning. On the contrary, you can celebrate right from the start... and continue celebrating for the rest of your life, rejoicing every time the thought of that evil monster enters your mind.

So get it perfectly clear in your mind: vaping is not your friend and never has been. Nicotine in any form is not your friend and never has been. It has done absolutely nothing for you, ever, other than harmed you constantly since the day you first started. It is your worst enemy and you are sacrificing nothing by cutting it out of your life, but just making marvellous positive gains.

So if you're wondering when the craving will go, the simple truth is:

THE CRAVING GOES WHENEVER YOU CHOOSE

You could spend the next few days, and possibly the rest of your life, continuing to believe that vaping or another form of nicotine was your friend and wondering when you'll stop grieving for it. Do that and you'll feel miserable, the craving may never go and you'll either feel deprived for the rest of your life or, more likely, you'll end up addicted to nicotine again and feeling even worse.

OR

You could recognise vaping and nicotine for the evil enemy that it really is. Then you need neither crave a vape or JUUL or IQOS or dip or snus or any other form of nicotine, nor wait for anything to happen. Instead, whenever the thought of vaping or nicotine enters your head, you can rejoice:

'YIPPEE! I'M FREE!'

REWIRE YOUR BRAIN

During the first few days after your final dose of nicotine, the Little Monster will be crying out, sending messages to your brain that it wants you to interpret as 'I want a vape'.

Now you understand the true picture, instead of feeling compelled to vape or feeling uptight because you can't, you know there's no need to panic. Pause for a moment, take a deep breath and simply brush the feeling away as if it were a piece of fluff on your shoulder.

Throughout this book you have been reprogramming your brain to enable you to see the true picture and to respond to the various triggers with a logical mindset, instead of the illogical, addicted mindset that you began with.

Previously your mind interpreted the withdrawal pangs of the Little Monster as 'I want a vape', because it had been filled with misinformation convincing it that a vape would satisfy the empty, insecure feeling. But now your brain is equipped with different information – the truth – and you understand that, far from relieving that feeling, nicotine caused it.

So just relax, keep your mind open and accept the feeling for what it is – the Little Monster fading away. In this frame of mind, these become moments of real pleasure rather than moments of struggle.

Now you need to prepare your mind for other triggers that may occur, particularly during the first few days after your final shot of nicotine. You might find, for example, that you forget you've quit. This can happen at any time. It often occurs first thing in the morning when you're coming around from sleep. You find yourself thinking: 'I'll get up and have a vape.' Then you remember that you've quit and you may feel shaken, worried that your mind is relapsing into the mindset of a vaper.

A similar thing may happen when you're socialising. Suddenly there's a JUUL or IQOS or mod thrust under your nose and you instinctively reach out to take it. Then you catch yourself and withdraw your hand. 'Aha!' say the vapers around you, 'I thought you'd quit.' They're almost gleeful, as if their main aim is to catch you out and drag you back into the trap.

Both of these situations can be disconcerting and doubts can creep in if you're not prepared, so make sure you're ready in advance. There will be times when you forget that you're a non-vaper and something will trigger your old thought process. This is actually a good sign. It shows that you're not obsessed with vaping or not vaping; you're just getting on with life like any other non-addict. It is not a sign that part of you still wants nicotine. Prepare yourself for these situations so you see them coming and are ready to remain calm and react with total confidence, laughing off your action and thinking: 'Isn't it great? I don't need to vape any more. I'm free!' These situations are no more concerning than taking the wrong turn to your old apartment shortly after you've moved.

Nicotine addicts will envy you because every single one of them would love to be like you.

FREE FROM THE NIGHTMARE

Other triggers could be after a meal, when having a drink, after making love... any of the occasions when you used to think vaping was 'special'. Although you have freed your mind from the illusion that these vaping moments were special, the association between these occasions and vaping can linger as a habitual reaction that turns your thoughts to nicotine. Again, see these moments as a cause for celebration. Rejoice that you are now able to enjoy and genuinely cherish these moments rather than interrupt the fun to have a vape and enslave yourself for life.

This interruption of relaxing moments (after a meal), social moments (with a drink), or moments of pure unbridled passion and pleasure (after love-making) occurs whether someone vapes or uses any other nicotine product. Being free from that is priceless. If your partner vapes – don't worry – cut them some slack and let them take their vaping breaks when they need to. Do your best not to make them feel bad about it and they'll see how easy you've found it to be free and will, in time, be likely to emulate you.

Once you're prepared, you won't be tripped up. Where you once had fear, you will have an incredible sense of freedom – the freedom of being a happy non-nicotine addict.

Chapter 17

TAKING CONTROL

IN THIS CHAPTER
•ONE SIMPLE STEP •WEAK EXCUSES
•ALL VAPERS WANT TO QUIT •BACK TO HEALTH

All vapers have their own powerful reasons for wanting to quit but they are afraid of what they're going to miss if they become a non-nicotine addict. When you quit, and realise you're not missing anything, you appreciate the greatest gain of all:

ESCAPE FROM THE SLAVERY

ONE SIMPLE STEP

Vapers start out with the belief that they are in control. Even after years in the trap, they still convince themselves that they do it because they enjoy it. Deep down, they know this isn't true, but they can't understand the real reason they continue to do it. It feels like an unseen force keeps compelling them to vape, even though they wish they didn't have to. That unseen force is fear created by addiction.

As I've explained, it is not a genuine fear – i.e., it is not based in reality and so it is not logical – but to the vaper it feels genuine enough. It is the fear of life being unbearable without nicotine. Nicotine addicts go through their entire addicted lives controlled by this fear, slaves to addiction. And because they don't understand it they close their minds to it and make up flimsy excuses for it – excuses like 'I like the taste' and 'It helps me relax' or 'It helps me concentrate'.

This is the Big Con that keeps all nicotine addicts in that miserable prison. It's an ingenious prison. It has no walls, no gates, no guards, nothing, yet the prisoners are kept captive by their own beliefs and fears, which are instilled in their minds by a tyrant called

ADDICTION

Not only does each prisoner act as their own jailer, they work together to keep everyone else imprisoned too, by spreading the fears instilled in them by the tyrant. Nobody knows exactly what would happen if they tried to escape, but they are sufficiently afraid of it to choose to stay in the prison, even though the tyrant has made it quite clear that he intends to imprison them and do them harm for the rest of their life.

They're so afraid of how bad things might get that they don't address how bad things already are.

Get this clear in your mind: nothing bad is happening here. You'll be missing out on nothing other than a lifetime of misery.

If you harbour slight doubts about nicotine helping you to be happy, helping you to cope with sadness or helping you to relax, concentrate, handle stress, enjoy a drink, enjoy a meal or make the most of a break from work, then see it the way it really is.

- **What does a nicotine addict *have to do* when they're happy?**

- **What does a nicotine addict *have to do* when they're sad?**

- What does a nicotine addict *have to do* when they want to relax?

- What does a nicotine addict *have to do* when they need to concentrate?

- What does a nicotine addict *have to do* if they need to handle stress?

- What does a nicotine addict *have to do* if they want to enjoy a drink?

- What does a nicotine addict *have to do* if they want to enjoy a meal?

- What does a nicotine addict *have to do* if they want to enjoy a break from work?

- What does a nicotine addict *have to do* after they make love?

Vapers have to vape. The same goes for JUULers, chewers and snusers. They do it because they are addicted to nicotine, and nicotine addiction steals their ability to make an informed choice.

They have to vape or JUUL or chew or snus day in, day out, every single day of their lives – never being allowed to stop.

They're incapable of doing anything without nicotine; either before, during or after.

The addiction makes it impossible for them to even grieve properly without nicotine. Can you think of anything more pathetic than that?

These aren't arguments for vaping or for nicotine; these are the biggest arguments against it.

THAT'S THE WAY IT IS

AND THE WAY IT ALWAYS WILL BE

Nothing will ever change the life of a nicotine addict. Except two things: stop living or

GET FREE!

There are evil regimes that have preyed on human fear throughout history. The tyrant of nicotine addiction is no less evil. But there is one key difference. If you had tried to escape the clutches of one of the tyrants the human race has thrown up so often, the consequences could have been dire.

Attempt to escape the clutches of nicotine addiction and nothing bad will happen to you at all. On the contrary, you will make many wonderful gains. You don't need to plot any daring escapes. There are no walls or fences to overcome, no guards training their guns on you. All you have to do is stop being controlled by the Big Con and step out of the prison.

It's that easy.

First of all, imagine being in that prison, crammed in with all the other nicotine addicts, all suffering, sick, enslaved and lying to yourselves and one another. Then imagine taking that one simple step to the outside, where the air is clean, your head is light and your vision is clear. That is the sense of freedom and happiness you can look forward to as a non-nicotine addict. That is freedom from slavery and it is the most wonderful of all the wonderful gains you stand to make by quitting nicotine.

WEAK EXCUSES

We all have our pride. Feeling controlled, like a slave, is a terrible blight on a person's self-esteem. All nicotine addicts suffer the indignity of having to see themselves as slaves and turn to a variety of phoney excuses in an attempt to promote an alternative explanation for their behaviour. After a short time in the trap the excuses change from deluded lies like 'I enjoy the taste' to defensive and negative arguments:

'I CAN AFFORD IT.'

You can probably afford to do all kinds of things but merely being able to afford something isn't an argument for doing it.

The thought of all the money you'll save when you get free won't help you to quit nicotine – but it certainly provides a great reason to be cheerful when you do.

'I HAVEN'T NOTICED ANY DETERIORATION IN MY HEALTH.'

So you're going to wait until you get ill before you consider quitting? Or are you denying that vaping is doing you harm? As a vaper, you instinctively know that you're doing yourself harm.

'I HAVEN'T GOT ANY OTHER VICES.'

So you're only vaping because you think you need a vice? That suggests you know it's bad for you, you're only doing it for that reason and you genuinely choose to do it. Where's the logic in that?

Drinking stagnant pond water is bad for you too. Why not 'choose' to do that instead? Or are you suggesting that vaping is more pleasant than drinking stagnant pond water? Really? How? At least pond water is free and it's not addictive. Would you drink pond water as a vice if it was flavoured with caramel? Of course not.

Drinking something is one thing, breathing it deep into your lungs is an entirely more serious matter.

Aside from the fact that these excuses have no foundation, they aren't so much reasons for vaping or being addicted to nicotine as reasons for not stopping. A double negative.

Compare that to the sort of reasons someone might give for taking part in a genuine pleasure, like taking part in a sport, going to the cinema or dancing.

'I enjoy the camaraderie.'
'I love the way it captures my imagination.'
'It transports me out of the present moment.'
'It makes me feel amazing.'

These are powerful, positive reasons for pursuing genuine pleasures, not weak excuses for not stopping doing them.

This highlights the difference between life as a nicotine addict and life as a non-nicotine addict. As a non-addict you don't need weak excuses. There is no sense that you're doing something so stupid that you need to justify it somehow. You can hold your head up high and speak the truth with enthusiasm and joy.

I'M A HAPPY NON-NICOTINE ADDICT. I'M FREE!

The Big Con keeps nicotine addicts trapped in prison by closing their minds to the truth. Easyway helps addicts take the easy step to freedom by opening their minds to the truth. And the simplest truth of all is this:

YOU DON'T NEED TO BE A SLAVE

Non-nicotine addicts who have never experienced addiction find it hard to understand why vapers need to have this simple truth pointed out to them. They have never been in the prison so they don't know what it's like in there. There are plenty of truths in life that are kept from us by industries that make gains from our ignorance: the junk food industry, for example. Plenty of non-nicotine addicts become obese by eating junk food. They too have missed a simple truth. They are no more or less stupid than vapers; if you're not told the truth, how are you supposed to know?

I was lucky enough to discover the simple truth that I took nicotine because I was addicted to it, not because I enjoyed it or derived some sort of crutch from it. Until that moment I had found it impossible to quit. That simple truth enabled me to walk free with one simple step.

Quitting nicotine means taking control and control comes with the realisation that you do have a choice. You don't need to remain a slave, you can walk free, you won't miss nicotine, you will enjoy life more, you will cope better with stress, you won't have to go through some terrible trauma to escape. This is the truth.

ALL VAPERS WANT TO QUIT

This is another truth concealed by the Big Con. All those poor souls in the prison secretly wish they could escape, but they don't admit it for fear of the consequences. If they admitted it, then they would have to go ahead and try to escape, and that prospect frightens them. They've been told that escape is painful and miserable at best, impossible at worst. So they keep their secret desire for freedom to themselves and carry on doing the tyrant's work, spreading the myth that they vape because they want to.

It's a fact that more and more vapers are now attending our seminars. They're either smoking and vaping or just vaping. If life as a vaper was that great, why would they pay us to seek our help? If you're a vaper and resistant to this argument, ask yourself why on earth you're reading this book. It's because you're fed up with the control and slavery of being an addict and simply want to be free.

Since the appearance of JUUL in the nicotine addiction market there is now a new generation of nicotine addicts who haven't ever smoked. Instead, they have exclusively used JUUL. The same with IQOS and whatever the latest nicotine delivery system is.

Whichever form of nicotine you're addicted to, even if it's multiple types, freedom from nicotine addiction is within your grasp right now. Take it.

Allen Carr's Easyway has grown into a worldwide phenomenon because of the universal demand among nicotine addicts for a cure that will help them to freedom. The vast majority of the people who attend our seminars around the world or read our books or use our online video programmes do so not as a result of advertising and marketing, but because they know an addict for whom the method worked. More often than not, they know many addicts for whom the method worked.

Every vaper or addict of any other nicotine product, either openly or secretly, would love to be in the position you'll be in when you finish this book. Most vapers are strong-willed and it frustrates them immensely that they can't gain control over their vaping. You are about to discover how wonderful it feels to be free from that frustration, that constant feeling of being controlled. It's a marvellous feeling, just to stand on the outside of that prison and look back at those poor nicotine addicts, not with envy or a sense of deprivation but with genuine pity, as you might look at any other drug addict. The greatest gain from being free is not so much the health gain or the money but the end of the self-loathing. You no longer despise yourself for being a slave to something you detest.

BACK TO HEALTH

The health risks of vaping and nicotine addiction aren't enough to motivate us to quit – but after your final dose of nicotine they became marvellous positive gains. The health scares cease to be a concern.

Non-nicotine addicts don't suffer any of the lows that nicotine addicts do. All this misery, all this fear, can be ended quickly, easily, painlessly and permanently by killing the Big Monster and stopping vaping or using nicotine in any form. No longer will you have to block your mind to health scares. Quite the opposite, in fact; you will rejoice in the feeling of your health being restored and protected.

Vapers often hide from the reality of the health scares – and perhaps you take the philosophical approach that we've all got to die some time so what's the point of worrying about it? Yet you worry about dying enough to look both ways before you cross the road, don't you? Your attitude isn't one of ignoring the bus hurtling towards you as you step off the pavement because 'Well, we've all got to go some time!', is it?

It's time to say goodbye to the worries of life as a nicotine addict once and for all. Let me turn that philosophical approach on its head:

if you never know how much life you have left, why spend that life burdened with unnecessary worries or even just the inconvenience of being addicted? Wouldn't it be better to enjoy every moment, free from worrying about your health and feeling like a slave?

Chapter 18

THE TRUTH ABOUT WITHDRAWAL

IN THIS CHAPTER

• *NO PAIN, HUGE GAIN* • *TRAUMATIC TALES FROM THE BIG CON*
• *NOTHING TO WAIT FOR* • *WITH EASYWAY, FREEDOM IS THE REWARD*

When nicotine addicts fear that quitting will be painful, they're thinking about the withdrawal period, when they first stop taking the drug and any remaining traces of it drain out of their system. They've been brainwashed to believe that the physical effects of withdrawal are traumatic. The truth is very different.

NO PAIN, HUGE GAIN

I've described the withdrawal from nicotine as a mild, uneasy, empty, slightly insecure feeling. I've also stated that the only reason a vaper or other nicotine addict takes the drug is to relieve that feeling, and that eventually that feeling causes a mental process during which the Big Monster creates the 'I want a vape! I can't have one! Aghhh!' feeling.

WITHDRAWAL IS 1 PER CENT PHYSICAL
AND 99 PER CENT MENTAL

The physical sensation of withdrawal is so mild as to be almost imperceptible. It doesn't matter even if you've been taking ridiculously high doses of nicotine – the feeling is very mild.

Vapers spend a lot of time planning to make sure they never find themselves in the dreaded situation of having no nicotine. It's a thought that can create panic long before they run out. How often have you been out at night and calculated that you'll be awake for another four hours, but only have enough nicotine left to last an hour? The realisation creates panic, which intensifies as you vape the last ration. Even though you're vaping and nicotine is flowing into your body, the panic feels like withdrawal pangs. That's the Big Monster.

THE PANIC-FREE VAPER

Most of the vapers and smokers who come to our seminars nod knowingly when I refer to 'that panic feeling' you get when you know your supply of nicotine is running out. But there's sometimes one who shows no recognition at all. 'I'm sorry,' he says, 'I have no idea what you're talking about.' The rest of the group stare at him in surprise.

Is he being honest? We know that all nicotine addicts have to lie to themselves, but when they come to one of our seminars we generally find that they welcome the chance to be honest and purge their conscience. So is the panic-free vaper or smoker the exception that proves the rule?

Not at all. The panic-free vaper or smoker is always a heavy user and the reason he doesn't know the panic feeling is because he has always made sure to avoid it. The panic-free addict is so frightened of suffering that panic feeling that he takes every precaution to make sure he never gets low on his drug.

And while he believes it must be his chosen brand or nothing, he has never tested that belief. The panic-free addict is neither lying nor telling the truth. He just hasn't discovered yet what it feels like to be denied his fix. Every nicotine addict who is prevented from taking their drug feels that panic.

The panic of withdrawal is all in the mind. It's the Big Monster that ties you in knots, makes you fidget and sends you racing to the shop in the middle of the night to make sure you're well stocked up. There is no physical pain. The physical sensation that arouses the Big Monster is minuscule.

It's uncertainty that causes the panic. Earlier we looked at the example of students sitting an exam without being distracted at all by the craving for nicotine. It's the same situation when you board a plane. You have certainty. You know you're not going to be allowed to vape for the next few hours so you stop worrying about it.

It's when you want a vape and feel you should be doing something about it that the fidgets start and the panic sets in.

We have spent some valuable time helping you to rewire your brain, clearing your mind of illusions and myths and replacing them with the certainty that nicotine does nothing for you whatsoever and you will not miss it at all. When you achieve that certainty about your decision to quit, the minuscule physical feeling of withdrawal doesn't induce fear and panic because you know exactly what's causing it and that it will be gone within a matter of days. The feeling is the Little Monster dying and you don't even have to wait until it's dead to start enjoying life as a happy non-nicotine addict. Whenever you feel that tiny sensation, rejoice in the knowledge that you're killing your mortal enemy and making your escape to freedom.

TRAUMATIC TALES FROM THE BIG CON

You have probably heard accounts from vapers who have tried to quit and reported that they went through some terrible trauma. You may even have suffered that trauma yourself. A quick internet search throws up a pretty unappealing list of the symptoms of nicotine withdrawal:

- **headaches**
- **coughing and sore throat**
- **nausea and intestinal cramping**
- **tingling hands and feet**
- **sweating**
- **weight gain**
- **anxiety**
- **irritability**
- **insomnia**
- **difficulty concentrating**
- **depression.**

Every one of these symptoms is a result of the mental panic that sets in when you try to quit with the willpower method. We've already discussed most of these symptoms, from weight gain down, and you should be clear that they are not caused by *not* vaping, they are caused by vaping. Depression, difficulty concentrating, insomnia, irritability, anxiety and weight gain are all psychological conditions. The first five symptoms are indeed physical but they are the physical manifestation of the intense stress that you put yourself under when you try to quit with willpower.

People who quit with willpower are taking a leap into the dark. They don't know what it takes to quit, let alone whether they have what it takes. They have no idea how long they'll need to draw on their willpower before their craving goes. They don't even know how they'll know whether they've succeeded in quitting or not. All this uncertainty is created by the belief that they're making a sacrifice. 'How long can I cope with feeling deprived?' No wonder they feel anxious as soon as they have their final dose of nicotine! They feel like they're jumping off a burning building with a blindfold on and waiting for the worst to happen.

It's the stress and anxiety that cause the headaches, nausea, sweats and other physical symptoms of withdrawal. Take away the stress and the physical symptoms go too. Be aware, too, that not every addict who quits with the willpower method suffers these symptoms. Most find that the withdrawal period is actually much less severe than they expected.

You're ahead of the pack – you already know that you have absolute certainty about what you're doing. By the time you begin to feel any slight physical feeling, you already know that you have no need or desire to vape again at any time in your life. The fact is you probably won't even notice any physical feelings. Certainly nothing more alarming than spotting a piece of fluff, out of the corner of your eye, on your shoulder.

'THAT'S ALL VERY WELL AND GOOD, BUT WHEN I QUIT IN THE PAST IT WAS TORTURE! HOW IS THAT NOT GOING TO HAPPEN AGAIN?'

That's a fair question, and it'll certainly help if you can understand what's happened in the past when you tried to quit and failed. Not only that, but this is part recap from earlier in the book, when I talked about having that 'I want a vape' thought.

It is also an explanation of how 'habit' and 'routine' can cause trigger moments WITHOUT causing you problems when you've quit.

What vapers suffer when they use willpower to stop are not physical withdrawal pangs from nicotine but feelings of deprivation, frustration and irritation resulting from a particular mental process. I'm now going to illustrate that mental process.

Let's see what happened to you in the past when you tried to stop vaping and failed. You failed because your brain became obsessed with nicotine and you felt terrible because of what you thought was nicotine withdrawal.

It starts with our routine. Now please don't misunderstand me. You don't vape because you're in the routine or habit of doing it. Habits are easy to break. For example, if you take a morning shower you might brush your teeth beforehand.

This would be a habit or routine that you will have repeated every day for many years without even thinking about it. If you wanted to change that habit and brush your teeth after your shower instead, would that be difficult? No, of course not.

You might find yourself reaching for the toothbrush before heading for the shower for the first few days. If so, that would easily be rectified by putting a sign by the toothbrush to remind you to shower first. After a couple of weeks, it would then become second nature and you'd have to make a conscious effort to change back if you wanted to. So a habit or routine which has become so ingrained that you've been doing it automatically every day for many years without even thinking about it, can be changed overnight without the slightest difficulty.

Our routine often triggers thoughts by association. Imagine that you tried to stop vaping in the past and your routine brought you back home from work in the evening.

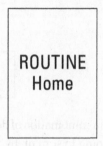

This might have been a moment in the past when you would have had a vape. It triggers a thought.

'I want a vape!' – let's call that 'IWAV'

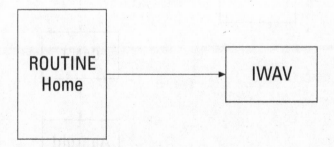

The next thought you have is: 'I CAN'T HAVE ONE.'

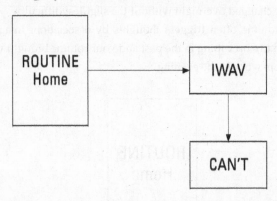

The next feeling you have is a combination of deprivation, frustration and irritation, which I'm going to sum up by the word 'Aaargh!'

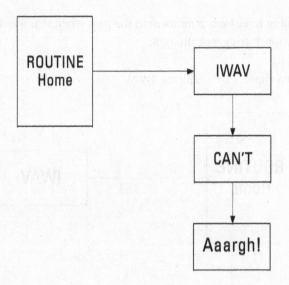

I can't explain it any better than 'Aaargh!'. It's a horrible feeling. Remember right now – the feeling wasn't triggered by nicotine withdrawal. It's the result of that 'IWAV' thought.

You now wind yourself up even more by telling yourself: 'I can't bear this, so I'll try not to think about it.' So you battle it and fight it and try not to think about it.

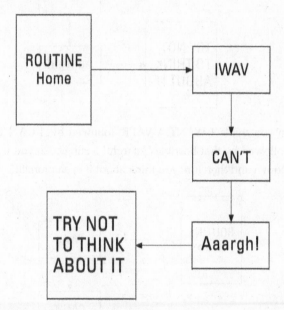

Then what happens? You think about it even more! It's impossible to force yourself to 'not think' about something. If I say, 'Whatever you do, don't think about a pink elephant now', what are you thinking about? Exactly – a pink elephant. By trying not to think about it, your brain becomes obsessed with it. Which once again triggers the 'IWAV' thought. And the cycle of misery, torture and hell speeds up.

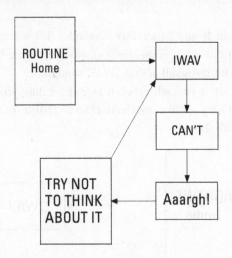

So again you think 'I WANT A VAPE' followed by 'I CAN'T HAVE ONE', followed by that horrible 'Aaargh!' feeling... so you try not to think about it and therefore you think about it even more!!!!

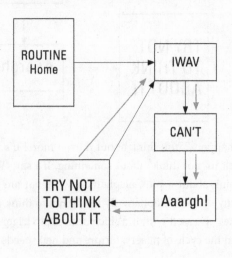

All you did was get home from work! This process is repeated at all the trigger moments you've battled with in the past when you tried to quit. After dinner, after leaving the Tube or getting off the bus, during a break from work, after making love. It can turn moments of real, genuine pleasure into moments of despair.

I'll stress this again. You need to realise that the 'Aaargh!' feeling is nothing to do with nicotine withdrawal. It's a feeling resulting from the mental process: 'I WANT A VAPE... I CAN'T HAVE ONE... Aaargh!'

Nicotine withdrawal was occurring during your Tube journey home from work – but it's so slight you weren't aware of it. As you step out of the Tube you automatically have a vape. You're responding to the very mild physical withdrawal and the fact that the withdrawal, combined with routine or habit, triggers the 'IWAV' thought.

It's the mental process that makes the withdrawal period insufferable.

UNLESS. YOU. GET. YOUR. HEAD. RIGHT!

Allen Carr's Easy Way to Quit Vaping effectively rewires your brain to disrupt those dysfunctional thought processes. It reboots your mind back to its natural state, before you became addicted to nicotine.

Rather than mistaking the physical reaction to a mental process for physical withdrawal from nicotine and having to battle it, you simply 'reboot', correct your thinking and feel great.

Thinking 'IWAV' really isn't a problem when you're a happy non-vaper.

Some people ask me how long before they won't think 'IWAV' at all. That varies, but the truth is it really doesn't matter as long as you are happy not vaping.

Have you ever rearranged the furniture in a room at home? You're delighted with the new layout and the way it looks. Later you walk back into the room and the new layout takes you a little by surprise. It takes a short, painless moment of adjustment to get used to the new layout. That might occur a few times over the first day or so – but very quickly the new layout becomes the complete norm.

The process certainly isn't unpleasant. In fact, it just reminds us that the layout of the room is now exactly as you wanted it.

The essential thing for you to understand at this point is what that 'I WANT A VAPE' thought means after you've finished this book.

Some people think it's obvious and say: 'Well if my brain thinks I WANT A VAPE, then it must mean that I WANT A VAPE!', but that's simply not true. At the height of an argument with a friend your brain might momentarily think: 'I could kill you now.'

That thought doesn't make you a murderer. It doesn't even mean that you're a bad person. It's just a thought. Rather than merely the thought being important, it's how you react to the thought that matters.

The human brain has tens of thousands of thoughts each day – so many that we can't even process them all. Some of them are wild and whacky. Some of them are completely inappropriate. You might be a perfectly normal person and you may well have had quite a few wild and whacky thoughts today already.

Let me give you an example. This is not a wild or whacky example, it's just an example of how your brain gets it wrong sometimes and also illustrates how we deal with that error without anxiety, concern or self-doubt.

Imagine you have your own designated parking spot at work or at home and you park your car there every day for a year.

Now imagine that your designated parking spot is moved just one space along the row. On the first day after the changeover would you be surprised if you parked your car in the old parking spot by mistake?

Of course not, it's almost bound to happen.

Now imagine that you do exactly that. You drive into the old parking spot by accident.

Would you turn the engine off, throw your hands in the air and say, 'My goodness, I'm SO infatuated with this parking space, I'm so emotionally attached to it, I can't possibly move'? Of course not!

What would you do? You'd simply move the car to the new parking spot.

Would you start worrying that you've got a car-parking problem? Of course not.

Does it mean that you desperately want to park in your old parking spot rather than the new one? Of course not.

So what does it mean?

It just means that your brain forgot that your parking spot had moved. That's all. And it's not a big deal.

If the same thing happened again the next day, it wouldn't bother you either. You would just re-park your car. It wouldn't take any willpower, and it doesn't mean that you want to park in one spot rather than the other. It just means that your brain needs a little time to automatically log that your parking spot has moved. It's very basic rewiring.

You've put a ton of metal in the wrong spot and you just brush it off without any self-doubt or recrimination. In fact, can you imagine the physical feeling you'd get as you realised you'd just pulled into the wrong spot? A slight tightness, a feeling in your gut. That's exactly the same feeling as the 'I WANT A VAPE' feeling, but because you brush it off automatically it doesn't fester, and develop, and grow into 'Aaargh'. If you understand how this could happen in the example of parking your car in the same spot, once a day, every day, for one year –

think about how many times a day as a vaper or JUULer or IQOSer or dipper or chewer or snuser you might have that IWAV thought.

I guess in the case of JUUL it would be IWAJ! And so on.

You get the point. You have that thought ten, twenty, fifty or even hundreds of times a day, and it's not something you've been thinking and reacting to for just a year, but for how many years?

Do you understand, just on principle, that after you complete this book, the thought 'IWAV' doesn't mean that you actually want a vape?

Of course it doesn't – it just means that for a moment your brain has forgotten that you've quit, which after years of vaping isn't surprising.

You don't want to be addicted to nicotine any more. You definitely don't want to vape, or JUUL or dip or chew or whatever. That's why you're reading this book.

So, if that 'IWAV' or 'IWAJ' or whatever 'IWA-thought' pops into your mind once you've quit, and it momentarily triggers the 'Aaargh' feeling, don't panic. Be cool, welcome it, rebalance yourself and think: 'YIPPEE – I'm free!'

It's only when you try not to think about it that it causes a problem. When you remind yourself about the parking space analogy, you won't be able to stop smiling.

Rather than having moments of struggle or upset, which creates a horrible negative cycle, you'll experience moments of pure joy.
If you can understand all I've said just on principle, then your brain is halfway home to being rewired and rebooted already.

Your reaction to 'Aaargh' won't be to try not to think about it, therefore ensuring that you think about it even more. Instead your reaction will be to reboot, correct and feel great.

When you had nicotine for the first time, you created an evil Little

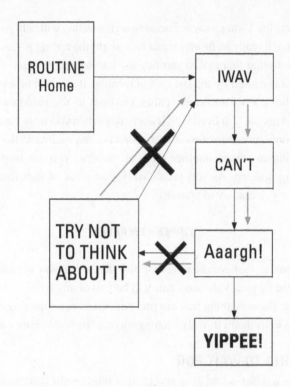

Monster inside your body, a parasite that feeds on a powerful poison called nicotine. As soon as you stop letting nicotine into your body and cut off the Little Monster's supply of nicotine, you have done the one thing required to purge yourself of that evil monster.

From this moment the Little Monster begins to die. In its death throes it will try to entice you to feed it. Create a picture in your mind of this vile little parasite writhing and squirming and enjoy starving it to death.

Keep this image in mind and you will ensure that you don't mistake the feeling for 'I want a vape'. Focusing on the feeling will help you to see it for what it really is. Be aware just how slight the feeling is – an empty, insecure feeling that makes you fidget a bit. Remind yourself that this feeling was caused by the last shot of nicotine. It may not be a pleasant feeling but it's not intolerable either. Far from it. You could easily live with it. After all, you lived with it every day when you were vaping.

The only difference now is that instead of responding to the feeling by vaping or taking another form of nicotine, you are responding by doing nothing. As you brush away that piece of fluff from your shoulder you can say to yourself:

'YIPPEE – I'M FREE!'

The monster that would have happily destroyed you is now being destroyed *by* you. Very soon you will be free of any trace of the Little Monster. The only thing that can prevent that from happening is if you respond to its death throes by letting nicotine back into your body.

NOTHING TO WAIT FOR

Nicotine is a fast-acting drug and most of it leaves the body in a matter of hours. However, you might be aware of the final traces of it leaving your body for a few days.

For those who quit with willpower, the period after the Little Monster dies can be a dangerous time. Having started out obsessed with not being allowed to vape, they suddenly realise that time has gone by and they haven't thought about vaping. This typically happens after about three weeks, or just over a couple of weeks after the end of the withdrawal period.

Everything the vaper hoped for appears to have come true. They have managed to go three weeks without doing it and it seems they're not even missing it. Wow! It wasn't that hard after all. This is cause for a small reward. And what possible harm could it do to reward themselves with just one vape?

If they're foolish enough to have one, they'll find themselves back in the trap in no time at all.

The fact that the vape does nothing for them gives them extra confidence. But they've put nicotine back into their body and soon they will feel the withdrawal symptoms again. One little voice will be saying: 'I don't want to vape', but another will be saying: 'Maybe, but I'd like another one.' They'll exercise their self-control and resist having another one immediately. They don't want to end up on the hook again, so they allow some time to pass.

They feel like they're in complete control, but already their willpower is being undermined. The next time they're tempted they can now tell themselves: 'I vaped last time and didn't get hooked, so what's the harm in having another?'

Ring any bells?

Before long they're right back in the trap, cursing themselves for their weakness and resigning themselves to a lifetime of addiction.

The fact is, most people who use willpower to quit experience discomfort for months afterwards. They might have killed the Little Monster, but the Big Monster is what causes all the unpleasant symptoms. It is their response to a thought process that is no longer triggered by nicotine withdrawal, but by something reminding them that they used to vape.

People who quit with the willpower method are always watching the clock, always chalking off the days, always feeling like they deserve a reward. With Easyway, there's no sense of marking time and no need for a reward, because you don't feel as if you're depriving yourself of anything. In fact, you're rewarding yourself from the moment you finish your final dose of nicotine.

WITH EASYWAY, FREEDOM IS THE REWARD

So by the time the Little Monster dies, you will already be getting on with life as a happy non-vaper and you probably won't even notice the withdrawal symptoms, let alone the fact that they've stopped.

The point is that there is absolutely nothing to fear from the withdrawal period after you quit. You don't have to wait to get through it or behave any differently when it's over. In fact:

ENJOY IT!

Soon you will have your final shot of nicotine ever. The thought of this moment and the freedom from nicotine addiction is incredibly exciting and the thrill can make you feel jittery, nervous and impatient. You might mistake these feelings for panic but you can easily dispel any confusion by reminding yourself of everything you know and understand and asking yourself what possible reason you have to panic. Nothing bad can happen by stopping vaping. Only good can come of it.

Be aware of your reasons for feeling so excited. The tyrant of nicotine addiction has dogged you for too long and now you are about to be rid of it. You have unravelled all the brainwashing that kept you imprisoned and miserable and very soon you are going to complete the simple step to freedom. From then on you will start to feel physically and mentally stronger. You will have more money, more energy, more confidence and more self-respect.

You stand on the brink of a magnificent achievement. Has it been hard getting to this point? Have you found it painful? Or are you now convinced that it is possible to quit vaping easily, painlessly and permanently, without relying on willpower or using substitutes?

If so, you're ready to prepare yourself for the ritual of

THE FINAL DOSE OF NICOTINE

Chapter 19

YOUR FINAL DOSE OF NICOTINE

IN THIS CHAPTER

•WHY ARE YOU DOING THIS? •CHOOSE YOUR MOMENT
•YOUR CHECKLIST

And so the moment has arrived. You stand on the brink of becoming a happy non-nicotine addict – completely free from nicotine – a marvellous achievement that will bring you tremendous benefits. All that's left is for you to complete the ritual of the final dose of nicotine. I'll specifically instruct you exactly when you should do that.

WHY ARE YOU DOING THIS?

That may strike you as an odd question at this late stage, but it's a question many nicotine addicts ask themselves as they face the prospect of having their last dose. It's important to check that you are quitting for the right reason. There are many good reasons for getting free from nicotine – health, money and guilt about your loved ones and dependants, for example – but these reasons alone are not enough. If they were, nobody would continue to take nicotine. You need to be clear that you are quitting because...

THERE IS ABSOLUTELY NO REASON TO CONTINUE
TO TAKE NICOTINE IN ANY FORM

To the non-nicotine addict, this statement seems glaringly obvious, but for nicotine addicts it's possible to go through life without ever realising this simple truth: that nicotine does nothing for you; it gives you no genuine pleasure or crutch; and you will not miss it. Allen Carr's Easyway has changed the lives of tens of millions of nicotine addicts by opening their eyes to the reality of the situation. When the penny drops, the feeling of relief is fantastic.

It is also essential that you have not made the decision to quit for the benefit of someone else. Many vapers say they want to quit for the sake of their children or their partner. If you do that you will feel that you are depriving yourself, and sooner or later you will be tempted to 'reward' yourself with just one vape or vape after an argument with them in a petty act of defiance. That one will be enough to set the whole vicious circle in motion again.

You are quitting for the best reason of all: your own happiness. It's you who are getting free, you who are rediscovering the genuine pleasures in life, you who are shaking off the shackles of slavery. As a nicotine addict you lose your grasp of many of the feelings that make life a joy: feeling healthy, energetic, guilt-free, unstressed, in control, happy. As a non-nicotine addict you will rediscover all these feelings and you will wonder how you ever feared life without nicotine.

EIGHTH INSTRUCTION: DO IT FOR YOURSELF, NOT ANYONE ELSE

Quit for the simple, selfish reason that you'll simply enjoy life so much more as a non-nicotine addict. All the other specific things involved –

the health benefits, release from the slavery, saving of money, freedom from guilt and fear and the pleasure and relief that your loved ones will feel – are just fabulous extra bonuses for you to enjoy.

Nicotine traps you in the slavery of addiction. It twists your perception of reality and fills your head with myths and illusions that keep you in the trap. Freedom is joyful.

There are no thrills to be had from nicotine. There is no pleasure at all; it was all just a confidence trick.

Happily for you, you have found an easy way to quit – you've found EASYWAY.

You are now equipped with all the knowledge you need to escape from the nicotine trap easily, painlessly and permanently.

CHOOSE YOUR MOMENT

A lot of people reach this point in the method feeling that they already have no need or desire to ever take nicotine again and ask whether it's essential for them to go through the ritual of the final dose. If you don't feel that way, don't worry, even if you feel sceptical. You're in for a fabulous surprise.

The ritual is important.

This is a momentous occasion, a huge achievement in your life and one that you will always look back on with a sense of pride and elation. It's important to mark the occasion indelibly. The dose of nicotine is your opportunity to focus one last time on the vile reality of nicotine addiction and then draw a line under it. That said, if you haven't taken nicotine for a few days, there is no need for you to go through this ritual. Just confirm to yourself that you've already taken your final dose of nicotine when I prompt you to have your final dose, and vow never to let it enter your body again.

So all that's left is for you to choose your moment. You may not have realised it, but you chose your moment when you bought this book. It will enable you to make the transition from unhappy nicotine addict to happy non-nicotine addict. All you need to do is finish the job.

ARE YOU READY NOW?

Of course you are – when you picked up this book you made the decision that you would become – or at least hoped to become – a non-nicotine addict. In fact you're all set to be a HAPPY non-nicotine addict.

That time has arrived. There is no reason to put it off.

This time, right now, is right for you.

Most attempts to quit vaping are timed to coincide with a particular occasion. New Year's Day is the classic example. New Year, new start. Sadly, attempts to quit on New Year's Day have the lowest success rate of any specific day.

Have you ever tried quitting on New Year's Day? You've vaped so much over Christmas that you're feeling sick of it. Your motivation to quit is high and the New Year seems like the perfect time to make a clean start. So you go through the ceremony of having your final vape as the clock strikes midnight on New Year's Eve.

So far, so good, but then a few days pass by and the excesses of Christmas are forgotten about. Your health has improved because of your abstinence from nicotine, but the Little Monster is crying out for its fix. The motivation for not vaping has gone, you're feeling strong and because you don't understand that nicotine will do nothing but guarantee the fidgets keep returning, you have a vape. Then you do it again and again and again.

Specific days like New Year's Day or a birthday are meaningless when it comes to quitting. They crystallise the motivation to quit, but the effect doesn't last. The feeling of deprivation replaces the desire to quit and we soon find ourselves making excuses to do it again. Having started again we're left with a miserable sense of failure and a reinforced belief that quitting is hard.

If you just so happen to be reading this book at New Year or on your birthday, please don't worry... you have the benefit of Easyway and in spite of, rather than because of, New Year or your birthday you'll find it easy to quit. Our intention here is to ensure that nicotine addicts don't delay quitting until one of those days rather than necessarily suggest that they avoid them.

Then there are those occasions that we had always told ourselves would be our cue to quit, like a health scare. The shock is often enough to make us bin vaping immediately, but after the initial shock comes the stress and anxiety, two feelings that typically drive us to our little crutch. As long as you believe that nicotine will help to relieve your anxiety and stress, it's inevitable that you will take it again before long.

Some nicotine addicts choose a time when they can get away from the usual temptations, such as their annual holiday or a quiet time on the social calendar. The trouble with this approach is that it leaves a lingering doubt: 'OK, I've coped so far but what about when I get back into the usual routine?'

If finishing this book just happens to coincide with one of the 'special days' I've mentioned above, don't worry; you'll succeed in spite of that, rather than because of it.

You need to be certain that you have no need or desire to take nicotine whatever the circumstances. Don't change your lifestyle: go out and enjoy social occasions, enjoy meals and handle stress from the start. When you've killed the Big Monster you have no need to give yourself time to adjust. You can start enjoying life as a happy non-nicotine addict the moment you finish your final dose.

You made the decision to quit nicotine the moment you purchased this book.

The time has come.

YOUR TIME TO STOP IS NOW – JUST A FEW MOMENTS AWAY

YOUR CHECKLIST

I'm sure that you have absolute certainty about your reason to quit and about the truth that there is no reason whatsoever to continue vaping or using nicotine in any form. You may not yet be able to imagine just how great you're going to feel when you get free but you should be feeling the excitement of something marvellous about to happen, like a parachute jumper standing in the open door of the plane. The wonderful truth is, there isn't even an ounce of danger in this instance.

A few butterflies are completely understandable. You are taking a big leap but you're not leaping blind. You are completely certain that what you're leaving behind is nothing but misery, degradation, filth and slavery. I can assure you that the feeling once you've stepped out towards freedom is nothing short of incredible. Nothing bad is going to happen; only a marvellous, exhilarating taste of freedom.

As a final confirmation that you're completely ready – let's use this checklist.

RATIONALISED

R Rejoice!
This is a momentous day. There is nothing to give up but there are many marvellous gains to make.

A Advice
Nicotine addicts offer it all the time. Ignore it if it conflicts with anything you've learned in this book.

T Timing
Why wait to get free? The ideal time to quit is now.

I Immediate
There is nothing to wait for when you quit with Easyway. You become a happy non-nicotine addict the instant you finish your final dose of nicotine.

O One Vape
There is no such thing as 'just the one'. One dose of nicotine is all it takes to drag you back into the nicotine trap.

N Never Again
This is the absolute end of your addiction. Never again will you feel the need or desire to vape or take nicotine in any form.

A Addictive Personality
Even if you had one, you became an addict because you took an addictive drug. You can just as easily become a non-addict.

L Lifestyle
There is no need to change it to avoid vaping situations, so do what you normally do when you normally do it.

I Intake
Never again subject your body to anything containing nicotine. The drug is the tyrant – how you take it is irrelevant.

S Sacrifice is Zero
There is nothing you're missing out on.

E Elephants
There's no need to avoid thinking about nicotine. Try to shut your mind to it and it will become your obsession.

D Doubt
Have none. You are making the most rational decision you've ever made.

Use the word 'RATIONALISED' to remind yourself of everything you know so that you never doubt your decision to quit and never again succumb to the feeling of 'I want a vape'.

NINTH INSTRUCTION: I WOULD NOW LIKE YOU TO HAVE YOUR FINAL DOSE OF NICOTINE PLEASE

Have your vape one last time. The same goes for snus, dip or any nicotine product – relate what I say now to those items accordingly.

What does the nicotine product look and feel like as you take it out of the packet? And how do you feel? Hold the nicotine product under your nose and take notice of how you feel as you sniff it. How is your heartbeat?

Continue applying this level of attention as you take your final dose. How does it smell? How does it taste?

What is the sensation on your tongue? In your throat? In your nose? In your lungs? How are you feeling?

This is one of those rare occasions in life when you are losing nothing and gaining so much. There is no price to pay for this joy and you won't feel any deprivation because you're not 'giving up' anything. You're ridding yourself of a deadly enemy. So rejoice.

As you finish your final dose close your eyes and make a solemn vow, a commitment to yourself, that you will never let nicotine into your body again.

Hold that thought. Never again will you have to subject yourself to this degradation.

Once you have done that, remove all traces of nicotine and nicotine devices. Throw them out immediately. You won't need them any more.

You can get on with your life as normal. With the added bonus of

FEELING INCREDIBLE

Chapter 20

STAY FREE

IN THIS CHAPTER
•FINALLY •CONGRATULATIONS!

Congratulations! You are now a happy non-nicotine addict! As you begin your new life, these simple tips will help to ensure you are never tricked into falling back into the trap. Don't wait for anything. You are already a non-addict. You became one the moment you finished that final dose of nicotine. You've cut off the supply of nicotine and unlocked the door of your prison.

Don't let a bad day at work or an argument with your partner break your stride
Accept that while it will have nothing to do with having quit nicotine, you will have good days and bad days. That's all part of the stresses and strains of life. However, because you will be stronger physically and mentally, you'll enjoy the good times more and handle the bad times better. Don't ever be tempted to blame a bad day at work or with your partner or the kids on the fact that you've quit nicotine.

Enjoy noticing the differences
Be aware that a very important change has happened in your life. Like all major changes, especially those for the better, it can take time for your mind and body to adjust. If you feel different or disorientated for

a few days, there's no need to worry. Just accept it. Feel it. A sense of quiet. A sense of peace. It might seem a little weird for a while. Have you ever seen a film when someone has been released from a dark, dismal dungeon? As they emerge into the bright sunshine, and feel the breeze on their cheek, they shield their eyes for a moment. Eventually they stop squinting, open their eyes and sense their freedom. This is where you are. Enjoy it.

Get out and enjoy life right from the start
You've quit nicotine, you haven't quit living. On the contrary, you can now start enjoying life to the full. Don't alter your lifestyle in any other way, unless you want to anyway. Carry on taking your breaks from work – take 'non-vape' breaks. Why miss out on the gossip and the chat of the smoking or vaping area just because you quit?

Don't avoid friends who smoke or vape
Do not try to avoid smokers or vapers. Go out and enjoy social occasions and handle stress right from the start. If your partner or best friend is a nicotine addict, don't avoid them, don't preach to them and don't interfere with their vaping or smoking. You've been released from a terrible ordeal – have compassion. Soon they'll see how cool, calm and collected you are about the whole thing, their curiosity will eventually overcome their fear of stopping and they'll be tempted into emulating you.

You don't need to quit drinking
In the past, when you tried to quit nicotine you may have lost your resolve after having a few drinks. That's what normally happens with the willpower method. If you're hanging on for grim life, a couple of

drinks loosens that grip. For this reason, with the best of intentions, people who attempt to quit nicotine sometimes also decide to quit drinking for a period as well. You simply don't need to do that. Don't start drinking if you don't drink already – but just do what you normally do, when you normally do it. If you normally go out for a drink on a Friday night – carry on doing so.

Never envy nicotine addicts
When you're with them remember that you're not being deprived, they are. They will be envying you because they will be wishing they could be like you:

FREE

Don't use substitutes
Forget substitutes or taking nicotine in any other form. You don't need them and they just keep people addicted to nicotine. Even apparently harmless substitutes, such as chewing gum or eating carrot sticks or sweets, will cause a problem. You don't need a substitute – you've got rid of a disease, not given something up. Any substitute can create and perpetuate a feeling of deprivation and soon awakens the Big Monster. Enjoy and cherish your freedom without substitutes.

Never doubt your decision
Never be in any doubt over your decision to quit – you know it's the right one. If you find yourself thinking: 'I want a vape', don't panic. Remember the parking space analogy. The feeling is just an echo from your nicotine-addicted days. That's a wonderful moment to remind yourself how lucky you are to be free. A moment when you brush that

piece of fluff off your shoulder and smile and enjoy the death throes of the Little Monster.

Remember, there is no such thing as 'one dose'
Be prepared for the offer of 'just one hit' or 'just one puff' from a friend, a colleague or even a stranger. Keep in mind that one dose of nicotine in any form is enough to drag you back into the nicotine trap. Remind yourself that you have no need for it and if you're offered 'just the one', remember, there is no such thing as one. See reality, which is a lifetime's chain of filth, disease and misery. See a hundred thousand doses – because…

THERE IS NO SUCH THING AS 'ONE'

Get rid of your device and leftover nicotine
Never keep any nicotine device or any nicotine with you or keep them anywhere in your house. If you do, you open the door to doubt and almost certainly guarantee failure. Would you advise an alcoholic to carry a flask of whisky in his pocket? That said, if your partner vapes, don't view this as a problem; you don't need to ban their nicotine sources from the house. Understand that there's a huge psychological difference between them keeping their nicotine in the house and you retaining some of yours. Get rid of yours; that's all you need to do.

Don't try 'not to' think about vaping or nicotine
Don't try to block the thought of nicotine from your mind. It's impossible to make yourself not think about something. By trying to you will make yourself frustrated and miserable. The thought of nicotine doesn't have to make you miserable; in fact, it should be a source of great joy. Instead

of allowing your thoughts to stray in the direction of 'I mustn't have a vape' or 'I can't have one', remember how lucky you are to be free.

'YIPPEE! I'M A NON-VAPER! I'M FREE!'

Make a written record
What was it about your life as a nicotine addict that made you want to quit? Write a page about it. Make sure you write it in the past tense. It is what you escaped from, so it must be in the past tense. Be sure to expand upon it also. For example, you could say, 'It controlled me'. But wouldn't it be more accurate to say, 'It controlled my life, what I did, when I did it and how I felt when I was doing it and that made me feel weak'. Go to town on this. Try to cover every aspect of your life as a nicotine addict and tell it exactly how it was.

Once you've done that for every aspect of your life as an addict, please keep that record to hand, in your handbag or your wallet, where you can take a look at it every now and then.

The idea isn't to be scared of going back to the addiction – it's a case of genuinely celebrating and cherishing your freedom.

Don't wait to become a non-nicotine addict
Don't wait for anything to happen. You don't need to wait to become a non-nicotine addict.

YOU ALREADY ARE ONE!

You became one the moment you went through the ritual of your final dose of nicotine.

FINALLY

What you have achieved is incredible – but remember, you are not alone. Tens of millions of nicotine addicts have quit with Easyway. Don't hold back from telling the world about your achievement. You won't be bragging; you'll be helping to dismantle the Big Con and will be doing your bit to enable and inspire tens of millions more addicts to escape to freedom and happiness.

If you ever have any doubts or concerns, or questions that arise, please don't hesitate to contact your nearest Allen Carr's Easyway centre. Every single one of our therapist teams around the globe quit nicotine with this method and they're always delighted to hear from anyone who has joined them in freedom or needs a little advice.

CONGRATULATIONS!

Lastly, congratulations on being free. Enjoy life, free from the nightmare – the life of a nicotine addict. It's been an absolute pleasure to guide you on your journey to freedom. Thank you.

ALLEN CARR'S EASYWAY CENTRES

The following list indicates the countries where Allen Carr's Easyway To Stop Smoking Centres are currently operational.

Check www.allencarr.com for latest additions to this list.

The success rate at the centres, based on the three-month money-back guarantee, is over 90 per cent.

Selected centres also offer sessions that deal with alcohol, other drugs and weight issues. Please check with your nearest centre, listed below, for details.

Allen Carr's Easyway guarantee that you will find it easy to stop at the centres or your money back.

JOIN US!

Allen Carr's Easyway Centres have spread throughout the world with incredible speed and success. Our global franchise network now covers more than 150 cities in over 45 countries. This amazing growth has been achieved entirely organically. Former addicts, just like you, were so impressed by the ease with which they stopped that they felt inspired to contact us to see how they could bring the method to their region.

If you feel the same, contact us for details on how to become an Allen Carr's Easyway To Stop Smoking or an Allen Carr's Easyway To Stop Drinking franchisee.

Email us at: join-us@allencarr.com including your full name, postal address and region of interest.

SUPPORT US!

No, don't send us money!

You have achieved something really marvellous. Every time we hear of someone escaping from the sinking ship, we get a feeling of enormous satisfaction.

It would give us great pleasure to hear that you have freed yourself from the slavery of addiction, so please visit the following web page where you can tell us of your success, inspire others to follow in your footsteps and hear about ways you can help to spread the word.

 www.allencarr.com/fanzone

You can "like" our Facebook page here **www.facebook.com/AllenCarr**

Together, we can help further Allen Carr's mission: to cure the world of addiction.

CENTRES

**LONDON CENTRE AND
WORLDWIDE HEAD OFFICE**
Park House, 14 Pepys Road,
Raynes Park, London SW20 8NH
Tel: +44 (0)20 8944 7761
Fax: +44 (0)20 8944 8619
Email: mail@allencarr.com
Website: www.allencarr.com
Therapists: John Dicey, Colleen
Dwyer, Crispin Hay, Emma Hudson,
Rob Fielding, Sam Kelser, Rob Groves,
Debbie Brewer-West, Duncan Bhaskaran-
Brown, Gerry Williams (Alcohol), Monique
Douglas (Weight)

Worldwide Press Office
Contact: John Dicey
Tel: +44 (0)7970 88 44 52
Email: media@allencarr.com

**UK Centre Information
and Central Booking Line**
Tel: 0800 389 2115 (UK only)

UK CENTRES
Birmingham
Tel & Fax: 0800 389 2115
Therapists: John Dicey, Colleen
Dwyer, Crispin Hay, Emma Hudson,
Rob Fielding, Sam Kelser, Rob Groves,
Debbie Brewer-West, Gerry Williams
(alcohol)
Email: mail@allencarr.com
Website: www.allencarr.com

Bournemouth
Tel: 0800 389 2115
Therapists: John Dicey, Colleen Dwyer,
Crispin Hay, Emma Hudson, Rob Fielding,
Sam Kelser, Rob Groves, Debbie Brewer-West
Email: mail@allencarr.com
Website: www.allencarr.com

Brentwood
Tel: 0800 389 2115
Therapists: John Dicey, Colleen Dwyer,
Crispin Hay, Emma Hudson, Rob Fielding,
Sam Kelser, Rob Groves, Debbie Brewer-West
Email: mail@allencarr.com
Website: www.allencarr.com

Brighton
Tel: 0800 389 2115
Therapists: John Dicey, Colleen Dwyer,
Crispin Hay, Emma Hudson, Rob Fielding,
Sam Kelser, Rob Groves, Debbie Brewer-West
Email: mail@allencarr.com
Website: www.allencarr.com

Bristol
Tel: 0800 389 2115
Therapists: John Dicey, Colleen Dwyer,
Crispin Hay, Emma Hudson, Rob Fielding,
Sam Kelser, Rob Groves, Debbie Brewer-West
Email: mail@allencarr.com
Website: www.allencarr.com

Cambridge
Tel: 0800 389 2115
Therapists: John Dicey, Colleen Dwyer,
Crispin Hay, Emma Hudson, Rob Fielding,
Sam Kelser, Rob Groves, Debbie Brewer-West
Email: mail@allencarr.com
Website: www.allencarr.com

Coventry
Tel: 0800 321 3007
Therapist: Rob Fielding

Email: info@easywaymidlands.co.uk
Website: www.allencarr.com

Cumbria
Tel: 0800 077 6187
Therapist: Mark Keen
Email: mark@easywaymanchester.co.uk
Website: www.allencarr.com

Derby
Tel: 0800 389 2115
Therapist: John Dicey, Colleen Dwyer,
Crispin Hay, Emma Hudson, Rob Fielding,
Sam Kelser, Rob Groves, Debbie Brewer-
West
Email: mail@allencarr.com
Website: www.allencarr.com

Guernsey
Tel: 0800 077 6187
Therapist: Mark Keen
Email: mark@easywaymanchester.co.uk
Website: www.allencarr.com

Isle of Man
Tel: 0800 077 6187
Therapist: Mark Keen
Email: mark@easywaymanchester.co.uk
Website: www.allencarr.com

Jersey
Tel: 0800 077 6187
Therapist: Mark Keen
Email: mark@easywaymanchester.co.uk
Website: www.allencarr.com

Kent
Tel: 0800 389 2115
Therapists: John Dicey, Colleen Dwyer,
Crispin Hay, Emma Hudson, Rob Fielding,
Sam Kelser, Rob Groves, Debbie Brewer-
West

Email: mail@allencarr.com
Website: www.allencarr.com

Lancashire
Tel: 0800 077 6187
Therapist: Mark Keen
Email: mark@easywaymanchester.co.uk
Website: www.allencarr.com

Leeds
Tel: 0800 077 6187
Therapist: Mark Keen
Email: mark@easywaymanchester.co.uk
Website: www.allencarr.com

Leicester
Tel: 0800 321 3007
Therapist: Rob Fielding
Email: info@easywaymidlands.co.uk
Website: www.allencarr.com

Lincoln
Tel: 0800 321 3007
Therapist: Rob Fielding
Email: info@easywaymidlands.co.uk
Website: www.allencarr.com

Liverpool
Tel: 0800 077 6187
Therapist: Mark Keen
Email: mark@easywaymanchester.co.uk
Website: www.allencarr.com

Manchester
Tel: 0800 077 6187
Therapist: Mark Keen
Email: mark@easywaymanchester.co.uk
Manchester—Alcohol sessions
Tel: +44 (0)7936 712942
Therapist: Mike Connolly
Email: info@stopdrinkingnorth.co.uk
Website: www.allencarr.com

Milton Keynes
Tel: 0800 389 2115
Therapists: John Dicey, Colleen Dwyer,
Crispin Hay, Emma Hudson, Rob Fielding,
Sam Kelser, Rob Groves, Debbie Brewer-
West
Email: mail@allencarr.com
Website: www.allencarr.com

Newcastle/North East
Tel: 0800 077 6187
Therapist: Mark Keen
Email: mark@easywaymanchester.co.uk
Website: www.allencarr.com

Northern Ireland/Belfast
Tel: 0800 077 6187
Therapist: Mark Keen
Email: mark@easywaymanchester.co.uk
Website: www.allencarr.com

Nottingham
Tel: 0800 389 2115
Therapist: John Dicey, Colleen Dwyer,
Crispin Hay, Emma Hudson, Rob Fielding,
Sam Kelser, Rob Groves, Debbie Brewer-
West
Email: mail@allencarr.com
Website: www.allencarr.com

Oxford
Tel: 0800 389 2115
Therapists: John Dicey, Colleen Dwyer,
Crispin Hay, Emma Hudson, Rob Fielding,
Sam Kelser, Rob Groves, Debbie Brewer-
West
Email: mail@allencarr.com
Website: www.allencarr.com

Reading
Tel: 0800 389 2115
Therapists: John Dicey, Colleen Dwyer,

Crispin Hay, Emma Hudson, Rob Fielding,
Sam Kelser, Rob Groves, Debbie Brewer-
West
Email: mail@allencarr.com
Website: www.allencarr.com

SCOTLAND
Glasgow and Edinburgh
Tel: +44 (0)131 449 7858
Therapists: Paul Melvin and Jim McCreadie
Email: info@easywayscotland.co.uk
Website: www.allencarr.com

Southampton
Tel: 0800 389 2115
Therapists: John Dicey, Colleen Dwyer,
Crispin Hay, Emma Hudson, Rob Fielding,
Sam Kelser, Rob Groves, Debbie Brewer-West
Email: mail@allencarr.com
Website: www.allencarr.com

Southport
Tel: 0800 077 6187
Therapist: Mark Keen
Email: mark@easywaymanchester.co.uk
Website: www.allencarr.com

Staines/Heathrow
Tel: 0800 389 2115
Therapists: John Dicey, Colleen Dwyer,
Crispin Hay, Emma Hudson, Rob Fielding,
Sam Kelser, Rob Groves, Debbie Brewer-West
Email: mail@allencarr.com
Website: www.allencarr.com

Stevenage
Tel: 0800 389 2115
Therapists: John Dicey, Colleen Dwyer,
Crispin Hay, Emma Hudson, Rob Fielding,
Sam Kelser, Rob Groves, Debbie Brewer-West
Email: mail@allencarr.com
Website: www.allencarr.com

Stoke
Tel: 0800 389 2115
Therapists: John Dicey, Colleen Dwyer,
Crispin Hay, Emma Hudson, Rob Fielding,
Sam Kelser, Rob Groves, Debbie Brewer-West
Email: mail@allencarr.com
Website: www.allencarr.com

Surrey
Park House, 14 Pepys Road, Raynes Park,
London SW20 8NH
Tel: +44 (0)20 8944 7761
Fax: +44 (0)20 8944 8619
Therapists: John Dicey, Colleen
Dwyer, Crispin Hay, Emma Hudson,
Rob Fielding, Sam Kelser, Rob Groves,
Debbie Brewer-West, Duncan Bhaskaran-
Brown, Gerry Williams (Alcohol), Monique
Douglas (Weight)
Email: mail@allencarr.com
Website: www.allencarr.com

Watford
Tel: 0800 389 2115
Therapists: John Dicey, Colleen Dwyer,
Crispin Hay, Emma Hudson, Rob Fielding,
Sam Kelser, Rob Groves, Debbie Brewer-
West
Email: mail@allencarr.com
Website: www.allencarr.com

Worcester
Tel: 0800 321 3007
Therapist: Rob Fielding
Email: info@easywaymidlands.co.uk
Website: www.allencarr.com

WORLDWIDE CENTRES

AUSTRALIA
ACT, NSW, NT, QSL, VIC
Tel: 1300 848 028

Therapists: Natalie Clays and Team
Email: natalie@allencarr.com.au
Website: www.allencarr.com

South Australia
Tel: 1300 848 028
Therapist: Jaime Reed
Email: sa@allencarr.com.au
Website: www.allencarr.com

Western Australia
Tel: 1300 848 028
Therapist: Natalie Clays and Team
Email: wa@allencarr.com.au
Website: www.allencarr.com

AUSTRIA
Sessions held throughout Austria
Freephone: 0800RAUCHEN
(0800 7282436)
Tel: +43 (0)3512 44755
Therapists: Erich Kellermann and Team
Email: info@allen-carr.at
Website: www.allencarr.com

BAHRAIN
Please check website for details
Website: www.allencarr.com

BELGIUM
Antwerp
Tel: +32 (0)3 281 6255
Fax: +32 (0)3 744 0608
Therapist: Dirk Nielandt
Email: info@allencarr.be
Website: www.allencarr.com

BRAZIL
Therapist: Lilian Brunstein
Email: lilian@easywaysp.com.br
Website: www.allencarr.com

BULGARIA
Tel: 0800 14104 / +359 899 88 99 07
Therapist: Rumyana Kostadinova
Email: rk@nepushaveche.com
Website: www.allencarr.com

CANADA
Sessions held throughout Canada
Email: mail@allencarr.com
Website: www.allencarr.com

CHILE
Tel: +56 2 4744587
Therapist: Claudia Sarmiento
Email: contacto@allencarr.cl
Website: www.allencarr.com

CYPRUS
Please check website for details.
Email: mail@allencarr.com
Website: www.allencarr.com

DENMARK
Sessions held throughout Denmark
Tel: +45 70267711
Therapist: Mette Fønss
Email: mette@easyway.dk
Website: www.allencarr.com

ESTONIA
Tel: +372 733 0044
Therapist: Henry Jakobson
Email: info@allencarr.ee
Website: www.allencarr.com

FINLAND
Tel: +358-(0)45 3544099
Therapist: Janne Ström
Email: info@allencarr.fi
Website: www.allencarr.com

FRANCE
Sessions held throughout France
Freephone: 0800 386387
Tel: +33 (4)91 33 54 55
Therapists: Erick Serre and Team
Email: info@allencarr.fr
Website: www.allencarr.com

GERMANY
Sessions held throughout Germany
Freephone: 08000RAUCHEN
(0800 07282436)
Tel: +49 (0) 8031 90190-0
Therapists: Erich Kellermann
and Team
Email: info@allen-carr.de
Website: www.allencarr.com

GREECE
Sessions held throughout Greece
Tel: +30 210 5224087
Therapist: Panos Tzouras
Email: panos@allencarr.gr
Website: www.allencarr.com

GUATEMALA
Tel: +502 2362 0000
Therapist: Michelle Binford
Email: info@dejadefumarfacil.com
Website: www.allencarr.com

HONG KONG
Email: info@easywayhongkong.com
Website: www.allencarr.com

HUNGARY
Sessions held throughout Hungary
Tel: 06 80 624 426 (freephone) or
+36 20 580 9244
Therapist: Gábor Szász
Email: szasz.gabor@allencarr.hu
Website: www.allencarr.com

INDIA
Bangalore and Chennai
Tel: +91 (0)80 4154 0624
Therapist: Suresh Shottam
Email: info@easywaytostopsmoking.co.in
Website: www.allencarr.com

IRAN—Tehran and Mashhad
Please check website for details
Website: www.allencarr.com

ISRAEL
Sessions held throughout Israel
Tel: +972 (0)3 6212525
Therapists: Ramy Romanovsky,
Orit Rozen
Email: info@allencarr.co.il
Website: www.allencarr.com

ITALY
Sessions held throughout Italy
Tel/Fax: +39 (0)2 7060 2438
Therapists: Francesca Cesati
and Team
Email: info@easywayitalia.com
Website: www.allencarr.com

JAPAN
Sessions held throughout Japan
www.allencarr.com

LEBANON
Tel: +961 1 791 5565
Therapist: Sadek El-Assaad
Email: info@AllenCarrEasyWay.me
Website: www.allencarr.com

MAURITIUS
Tel: +230 5727 5103
Therapist: Heidi Hoareau
Email: info@allencarr.mu
Website: www.allencarr.com

MEXICO
Sessions held throughout Mexico
Tel: +52 55 2623 0631
Therapists: Jorge Davo and Team
Email: info@allencarr-mexico.com
Website: www.allencarr.com

NETHERLANDS
Sessions held throughout the Netherlands
Allen Carr's Easyway
'stoppen met roken'
Tel: (+31)53 478 43 62 /
(+31)900 786 77 37
Email: info@allencarr.nl
Website: www.allencarr.com

NEW ZEALAND
North Island – Auckland
Tel: +64 (0) 0800 848 028
Therapists: Natalie Clays and Team
Email: natalie@allencarr.co.nz
Website: www.allencarr.com
South Island – Wellington and Christchurch
Tel: +64 (0) 0800 848 028
Therapists: Natalie Clays and Team
Email: natalie@allencarr.co.nz
South Island – Dunedin and Invercargill
Tel: +64 (0)27 4139 381
Therapist: Debbie Kinder
Email: easywaysouth@icloud.com
Website: www.allencarr.com

NORWAY
Therapist: Laila Thorsen
Please check website for details
Website: www.allencarr.com

PERU — Lima
Tel: +511 637 7310
Therapist: Luis Loranca
Email: lloranca@dejardefumaraltoque.com
Website: www.allencarr.com

POLAND
Sessions held throughout Poland
Tel: +48 (0)22 621 36 11
Therapist: Michael Kochon
Email: info@allen-carr.pl
Website: www.allencarr.com

POLAND – Alcohol seminars
Please check website for details
Website: www.allencarr.com

PORTUGAL
Oporto
Tel: +351 22 9958698
Therapist: Ria Slof
Email: info@comodeixardefumar.com
Website: www.allencarr.com

REPUBLIC OF IRELAND
Dublin
Tel: +353 (0)1 499 9010
Therapists: Paul Melvin, Jim McCreadie
Email: info@allencarr.ie
Website: www.allencarr.com

ROMANIA
Tel: +40 (0)7321 3 8383
Therapist: Cristina Nichita
Email: raspunsuri@allencarr.ro
Website: www.allencarr.com

RUSSIA
Allen Carr's Easyway to Stop Smoking
Live Seminars & Online Video Programme
Tel: +7 495 644 64 26
Freecall +7 (800) 250 6622
Therapist: Alexander Fomin
Email: info@allencarr.ru
Website: www.allencarr.com

Allen Carr's Easyway to Stop Drinking
Live Seminars & Online Video Programme
Tel: +8 (800) 302 80 68

+7 985 207 47 93
Therapist: Artem Kasyanov
Email: info@allencarrlife.ru
Website: www.allencarr.com

St Petersburg
Please check website for details
Website: www.allencarr.com

SAUDI ARABIA
Please check website for details
Website: www.allencarr.com

SERBIA
Belgrade
Tel: +381 (0)11 308 8686
Email: office@allencarr.co.rs
Website: www.allencarr.com

SINGAPORE
Tel: +65 62241450
Therapist: Pam Oei
Email: pam@allencarr.com.sg
Website: www.allencarr.com

SLOVENIA
Tel: 00386 (0)40 77 61 77
Therapist: Grega Server
Email: easyway@easyway.si
Website: www.allencarr.com

SOUTH AFRICA
Sessions held throughout South Africa
National Booking Line:
0861 100 200
Head Office: 15 Draper Square, Draper St,
Claremont 7708, Cape Town, Cape Town: Dr
Charles Nel
Tel: +27 (0)21 851 5883
Mobile: 083 600 5555
Therapists: Dr Charles Nel,
Malcolm Robinson and Team
Email: easyway@allencarr.co.za
Website: www.allencarr.com

SOUTH KOREA — Seoul
Tel: +82 (0)70 4227 1862
Therapist: Yousung Cha
Email: master@allencarr.co.kr
Website: www.allencarr.com

SPAIN
Tel: +34 910 05 29 99
Therapist: Luis Loranca
Email: informes@AllenCarrOfficial.es
Website: www.allencarr.com

SWEDEN
Tel: +46 70 695 6850
Therapists: Nina Ljungqvist,
Renée Johansson
Email: info@easyway.se
Website: www.allencarr.com

SWITZERLAND
Sessions held throughout Switzerland
Freephone: 0800RAUCHEN
(0800/728 2436)
Tel: +41 (0)52 383 3773
Fax: +41 (0)52 3833774
Therapists: Cyrill Argast and Team
For sessions in Suisse Romand
and Svizzera Italiana:
Tel: 0800 386 387
Email: info@allen-carr.ch
Website: www.allencarr.com

TURKEY
Sessions held throughout Turkey
Tel: +90 212 358 5307
Therapist: Emre Üstünuçar
Email: info@allencarr.com.tr
Website: www.allencarr.com

UNITED ARAB EMIRATES
Dubai and Abu Dhabi
Tel: +971 56 693 4000
Therapist: Sadek El-Assaad
Email: info@AllenCarrEasyWay.me
Website: www.allencarr.com

USA
Sessions held throughout the USA
Toll free: 855 440 3777
Email: support@usa.allencarr.com
Website: www.allencarr.com

New York
Toll free: 855 440 3777
Therapists: Natalie Clays and Team
Email: support@usa.allencarr.com
Website: www.allencarr.com

Los Angeles
Toll free: 855 440 3777
Therapists: Natalie Clays and Team
Email: support@usa.allencarr.com
Website: www.allencarr.com

Milwaukee (and South Wisconsin)
Tel: +1 262 770 1260
Therapist: Wayne Spaulding
Email: wayne@easywaywisconsin.com
Website: www.allencarr.com

OTHER ALLEN CARR PUBLICATIONS

Allen Carr's revolutionary Easyway method is available in a wide variety
of formats, including digitally as audiobooks and ebooks, and has been
successfully applied to a broad range of subjects.
For more information about Easyway publications, please visit
shop.allencarr.com

Easyway to Quit Smoking

Stop Smoking Now

Quit Smoking Boot Camp

Your Personal Stop Smoking Plan

The Illustrated Easy Way to Stop
Smoking

The Easy Way for Women to Stop
Smoking

The Illustrated Easy Way for Women to
Stop Smoking

Finally Free!

Smoking Sucks (Parent Guide with 16
page pull-out comic)

The Little Book of Quitting Smoking

How to Be a Happy Non-smoker

No More Ashtrays

How to Stop Your Child Smoking

The Only Way to Stop Smoking
Permanently

Stop Drinking Now

The Easy Way to Control Alcohol

Your Personal Stop Drinking Plan

The Illustrated Easy Way to Stop
Drinking

The Easy Way for Women to Stop
Drinking

No More Hangovers

The Easy Way to Mindfulness

Good Sugar Bad Sugar

The Easy Way to Quit Sugar

Lose Weight Now

The Easy Way for Women to Lose Weight

No More Diets

The Easy Way to Lose Weight

The Easy Way to Stop Gambling

No More Gambling

No More Worrying

Get Out of Debt Now

No More Debt

No More Fear of Flying

The Easy Way to Quit Caffeine

Packing It In The Easy Way (the autobiography)

Want Easyway on your **smartphone** or **tablet**?
Search for "Allen Carr" in your app store.

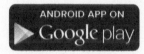 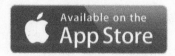

Easyway publications are also available as **audiobooks**.
Visit **shop.allencarr.com** to find out more.

 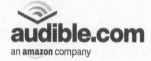

DISCOUNT VOUCHER
for
ALLEN CARR'S
EASYWAY CENTRES

Recover the price of this book when you attend an
Allen Carr's Easyway Centre
anywhere in the world!

Allen Carr's Easyway has a global network of stop
smoking centres where we guarantee you'll find it easy
to stop smoking or your money back.

**The success rate based on this
unique money-back guarantee is over 90%.**

Sessions addressing weight, alcohol and other
drug addictions are also available at certain centres.

When you book your session, mention this
voucher and you'll receive a discount of
the price of this book. Contact your nearest
centre for more information on how the sessions
work and to book your appointment.

**Details of Allen Carr's Easyway
Centres can be found at**
www.allencarr.com
or call 0800 389 2115

This offer is not valid in conjunction with any other offer/promotion.